HEAD AND NECK CANCER

A COMPREHENSIVE REVIEW OF HEAD AND NECK SQUAMOUS CELL CARCINOMA

DR. BHRATRI BHUSHAN
MBBS, MD (MEDICINE)
DM (MEDICAL ONCOLOGY)
CONSULTANT MEDICAL ONCOLOGIST AND HEMATOLOGIST

Copyright © 2019 by Dr. Bhratri Bhushan

All rights reserved. No part of this publication may be reproduced, distributed, or transmitted in any form or by any means, including photocopying, recording, or other electronic or mechanical methods, without the prior written permission of the publisher, except in the case of brief quotations embodied in critical reviews and certain other noncommercial uses permitted by copyright law. For permission requests, write to the publisher, addressed "Attention: Permissions Coordinator," at the address below.

A6, Jindal hospital, Hisar, Haryana, India
125001 www.bhratri@gmail.com

This work is provided "as is," and the author and the publisher disclaim any and all warranties, express or implied, including any warranties as to accuracy, comprehensiveness, or currency of the content of this work. This work is no substitute for individual patient assessment based on healthcare professionals' examination of each patient and consideration of, among other things, age, weight, gender, current or prior medical conditions, medication history, laboratory data, and other factors unique to the patient. The publisher does not provide medical advice or guidance, and this work is merely a reference tool. Healthcare professionals, and not the publisher, are solely responsible for the use of this work including all medical judgments and for any resulting diagnosis and treatments. Given continuous, rapid advances in medical science and health information, independent professional verification of medical diagnoses, indications, appropriate pharmaceutical selections and dosages, and treatment options should be made and healthcare professionals should consult a variety of sources. When prescribing medication, healthcare professionals are advised to consult the product information sheet (the manufacturer's package insert) accompanying each drug to verify, among other things, conditions of use, warnings, and side effects and identify any changes in dosage schedule or contraindications, particularly if the medication to be administered is new, infrequently used, or has a narrow therapeutic range. To the maximum extent permitted under applicable law, no responsibility is assumed by the publisher for any injury and/or damage to persons or property as a matter of products liability, negligence law or otherwise, or from any reference to or use by any person of this work.

CONTENTS

Title Page	1
Copyright	2
Dedication	5
CHAPTER 1: INTRODUCTION AND ETIOPATHOGENESIS	9
CHAPTER 2: PRINCIPLES OF PATHOLOGY	22
CHAPTER 3: CHEMOPREVENTION	38
CHAPTER 4: SCREENING	56
CHAPTER 5: PRINCIPLES OF DIAGNOSIS AND STAGING	68
CHAPTER 6: PRINCIPLES OF RADIATION THERAPY AND COMBINED CHEMORADIATION	81
CHAPTER 7: ORAL CAVITY	93
CHAPTER 8: OROPHARYNX	104
CHAPTER 9: HYPOPHARYNX	110
CHAPTER 10: LARYNX	113
CHAPTER 11: NASOPHARYNX	122

CHAPTER 12: SALIVARY GLAND TUMORS   127

CHAPTER 13: PARANASAL SINUSES, NASAL CAVITY AND NASAL VESTIBULE   134

CHAPTER 14: HEAD AND NECK CANCERS WITH DISTANT METASTASIS AND RECURRENCE   138

CHAPTER 15: SECOND PRIMARY MALIGNANCIES   144

CHAPTER 16: SURVIVORSHIP   147

"Success is not final, failure is not fatal: it is the courage to continue that counts."

WINSTON CHURCHILL

DR. BHRATRI BHUSHAN

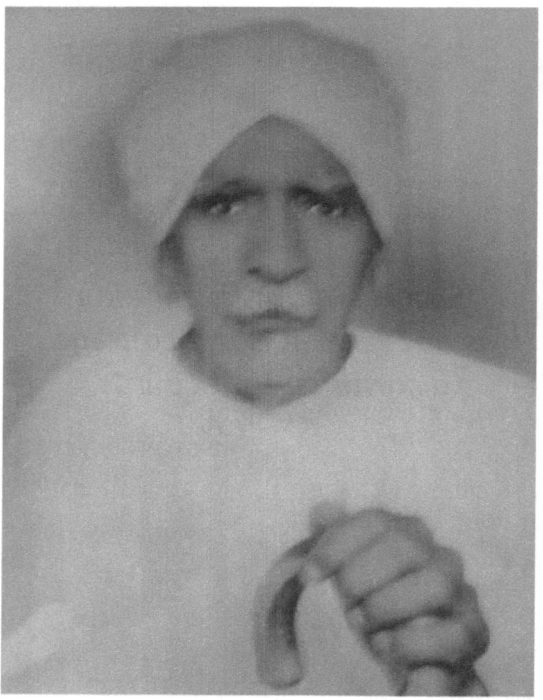

Dedicated to Pandit Sohanlal Arya (1900-1982); a revolutionary, a freedom fighter and above all, an epitomisation of honesty and probity incarnate. Who in the face of tyrannical British rule disseminated the light of knowledge and unified people for the cause. A grand scholar of Sanskrit and a visionary, great deeds of whom reverberate through to this moment and will continue to posterity.

PREFACE

Worldwide head and neck cancers occur in 550,000 people with around 300,000 deaths each year. Although head and neck region may give rise to many different histological types of malignancies, around 90% of all cancers affecting this region are squamous cell carcinomas. These are the sixth leading cancer by incidence worldwide.

Tobacco, smoked and smokeless, is the most important preventable risk factor. Alcohol is also a major independent risk factor, that when combined with tobacco has especially enhanced carcinogenic effects. More recently human papilloma virus (HPV) has emerged as a major etiology, especially for oropharyngeal carcinomas; affecting younger population, having better survival outcomes compared with cancers associated with tobacco and alcohol.

The five-year overall survival rate of patients with HNSCC, as a whole, is about 40-50%. About one third of patients present with early stage disease, while the rest are locoregionally advanced and metastatic.

This book encompasses head and neck cancers of squamous histology; ranging from epidemiology, risk factors, prevention, screening, diagnosis, treatment and survivorship; discussing each site separately and comprehensively but without in-depth analysis of the studies leading to these recommendations, to keep the reading succinct, uptodate and applicable to practice as well as informative for patients and general reading.

I am forever grateful to Godliness for bestowing upon me a fulfilling purpose to live, my family for being there always and my son Varchasv, for giving my life meaning.

CHAPTER 1: INTRODUCTION AND ETIOPATHOGENESIS

Head and neck cancers are the sixth most common malignancy worldwide, third most common in India and in some parts of India it's the most common malignancy. The anatomical structures encompassed in this broad term are oral cavity, paranasal sinuses, pharynx, larynx, cervical esophagus, thyroid, lymph nodes, soft tissues, and bone. This marked heterogeneity in the structures involved entails the possibility of development of myriads of cancer histologies.

A comprehensive anatomical review of all the structures in head and neck region is well beyond the scope of this book. Excluded from the discussion here are the cancers of thyroid glands, brain tumors and other rare neoplasms. A simple outline of the structures of head and neck, in accordance with the topics pertinent to the ensuing discussion in this book include one of the following five subsets: oral cavity (lips, buccal mucosa, anterior tongue, floor of the mouth, hard palate, and upper and lower gingiva); pharynx (nasopharynx, oropharynx, and hypopharynx); larynx (supraglottic, glottic, and subglottic regions); nasal cavity and paranasal sinuses (maxillary, ethmoid, sphenoid, and frontal) and salivary glands (parotid, submandibular, sublingual, and the minor glands).

The term "head and neck cancers" is used interchangeably with the histology *squamous cell carcinoma*, unless otherwise specified. The risk factors associated with these cancers are tobacco use in any form, alcohol consumption, human papillomavirus (HPV) infection (for oropharyngeal cancer), and Epstein-Barr virus (EBV) infection (for nasopharyngeal cancer). There are many other etiological agents as well, but they constitute causality in only a minority of cases.

Worldwide, head and neck cancer accounts for about 700,000 cases and half as many deaths per year. In the US around 50000 people develop head and neck cancers in a year, while 10000 succumb. Head and neck cancers are the third most common cancers in India with 52 067 deaths and 77 003 cases diagnosed in 2012. Particularly in India, the data mostly comes from tertiary care referral centres and the actual incidence and prevalence is certainly much higher. In Europe, there were approximately 250,000 cases (an estimated 4 percent of the cancer incidence) and 63,500 deaths in 2012.

Males are affected significantly more than females, the ratio being more than two to four times. There are regional variations as well, while larynx and pharynx cancers are the most common head and neck cancers in western world, in Indian subcontinent oral cavity cancers are more common and nasopharyngeal cancers are more prevalent in some Asian countries. These variations are due to the differences in predominant causative factors, for example smoking is more commonly implicated in larynx cancer while chewing tobacco results in more cases of oral cavity cancers.

Tobacco products use in form like smoking and chewing, is a very important and preventable cause of head and neck cancer. Many studies have been done on this subject, the estimated increase in the risk of developing head and neck cancer in cigarette smokers has been 5 to 25 fold. Not only the numbers of cigarettes smoked have the detrimental effects, but the age of starting to smoke and the total duration, as well as other contributory factors like concomitant alcohol consumption also have an influence on the attributed risk.

DR. BHRATRI BHUSHAN

The risk for HNSCC in smokers is approximately ten times higher than that of never smokers, and 70-80% of new HNSCC diagnoses are associated with tobacco and alcohol use. Tobacco products have been used for centuries; however, it is just within the last 60-70 years that we have developed an understanding of their damaging effects. This relatively recent understanding has created a pathway towards educational and regulatory efforts aimed at reducing tobacco use. Understanding the carcinogenic components of tobacco products and how they lead to HNSCC is critical to regulatory and harm reduction measures. To date, nitrosamines and other carcinogenic agents present in tobacco products have been associated with cancer development. The disruption of DNA structure through DNA adduct formation is felt to be a common mutagenic pathway of many carcinogens. Intense work pertaining to tobacco product constituents, tobacco use, and tobacco regulation has resulted in decreased use in some parts of the world. Still, much work remains as tobacco continues to impart significant harm and contribute to head and neck cancer development worldwide.

Other forms of smoking like pipes and cigars also cause head and neck cancers but large scale studies are lacking and the results are often confounded as it's difficult for a person to be only a cigar smoker and never having smoked a cigarette. Same holds true for chewable tobacco products. In one study, the risk in people who abused "smokeless" tobacco were found to at a four fold increased risk of developing head and neck cancer compared with never smokers.

The most important risk factor for developing head and neck cancer is tobacco with its effects linked to p53 mutations, alcohol and betel nut chewing have synergistic effect with tobacco. Tobacco smoke contains many known carcinogens of which benzo[a] pyrenediol epoxide, induces DNA adducts throughout the genome. These DNA damages are repaired by the human DNA repair machinery which includes nucleotide excision repair (NER) and base excision repair (BER) pathways. Genetic polymorphisms in the genes involved in NER such as ERCC-1 and XPD and in the genes involved in BER such as XRCC-1 and ADPRT may contribute to increased risk and susceptibility to head and neck squamous cell carcinoma (HNSCC).

Studies regarding the association between marijuana use and head and neck cancer have found conflicting results, partly because of the confounding factors like cigarette smoking and alcohol consumption, thus precluding a definitive result.

Alcohol has carcinogenic properties and has been

implicated in the development of many cancers including head and neck cancers; although in the latter case it's often not possible to separate the effects of alcohol from tobacco, the use of which often accompanies. Having said that, alcohol drinking is an established risk factor for head and neck cancers, and this association may be stronger among cancers of the oropharynx and hypopharynx than the oral cavity or larynx. In addition, higher alcohol consumption over a shorter period was more harmful than fewer alcohol consumption over a longer period, and the most frequently consumed alcoholic beverages in a population is likely to be associated with the highest risk of head and neck cancers in that population. The risk of head and neck cancers after ≥ 20 years of alcohol cessation appear to be similar to the risk among never drinkers. The interaction between genetic polymorphisms related to alcohol metabolism and alcohol drinking on the risk of HNC has been noted, and the prevalence of these genetic polymorphisms in each population should be of concern. On the other hand, the association between alcohol drinking and the survival of individuals with head and neck cancers remains unclear.

Many viral infections have been associated with an increased risk of head and neck cancer. The mechanism of development of head and neck cancer due to viral infections is incompletely understood. It has been demonstrated in studies that the viral genetic material influences certain key areas of host DNA and downstream genetic pathways, resulting in activation of oncogenes or inactivation of tumor suppressor genes.

Epstein-Barr virus is an established risk factor for the development of nasopharyngeal cancer throughout the world and especially in China. Epstein-Barr virus (EBV) is ubiquitous, over 90% of the adult population is infected with this virus. EBV is capable of infecting both B lymphocytes and epithelial cells throughout the body including the head and neck region. Transmission occurs mainly by exchange of saliva. The infection is asymptomatic or mild in children but, in adolescents and young adults, it causes infectious mononucleosis, a self-limiting disease characterized by lethargy, sore throat, fever and lymphadenopathy. Once established, the virus often remains latent and people become lifelong carriers without experiencing disease. However, in some people, the latent virus is capable of causing malignant tumours, such as nasopharyngeal carcinoma and various B- and T-cell lymphomas, at sites including the head, neck and oropharyngeal region.

Human papillomavirus has emerged as a major etiological agent in cancers of oropharynx. Until recently, approximately 20% of oral cancers and 60% to 80% of OPC were thought to be attributable to HPV infection. In 2012, the International Agency of Research of Cancer (IARC) declared that there was sufficient evidence to associate a subtype of HPV 16 with oral cancers. Epidemiologically, HPV-positive HNSCC occurs more frequently in younger patients (younger than 50 years), which differs from the typical age of HNSCC patients. A direct correlation between HPV-positive patients and sexual behavior has also been shown in HNSCC. High-risk HPV-16 is correlated with vaginal or oral sex and frequent sexual encounters without barrier usage. Current changes in sexual practices, including first sexual experience at an earlier age, high number of sexual partners, and high probability of oral sex, may be associated with the increasing prevalence of HPV infection.

Gene expression profiles also differ in HPV-positive oral cancers based on evidence from different pathways, such as the p53 and pRb pathways involved in cell cycling, the EGFR pathway, which is an important therapeutic target (especially in breast and lung cancers), the TGFβ pathway, the PI3K-PTEN-AKT pathway, and angiogenesis and hypoxia pathways. Sampling techniques for HPV include microscopy, ELISA, Southern blot, dot blot, hybrid capture, DNA microarray, and ligase chain reaction for probe amplification. Although a standard procedure has not yet been generally accepted, both polymerase chain reaction and *in situ* hybridization assays are well validated, and gene expression by DNA microarray has recently gained acceptance as a high throughput method.

HIV has been found to increase the incidence of head and neck cancer patients. This causality is incompletely elucidated and the overall immunodeficient state that results from HIV infection is thought more to contribute than the actual infection itself. Other immunodeficient state like those induced by solid organ transplantation protocols have also been linked to the increased incidence of head and neck cancers in the recipients.

Areca nut is the seed of the fruit of the oriental palm, *Areca catechu*. It is the basic ingredient of a variety of widely used chewed products. Thin slices of the nut, either natural or processed, may be mixed with a variety of substances including slaked lime (calcium hydroxide) and spices such as cardamom, coconut, and saffron. Most significantly, they may be mixed with tobacco products or wrapped in the leaf of the piper betel plant. Hence the more common name betel nut. Areca nut is used by an estimated 200-400 million people, mainly Indo-Asians and Chinese. It is used by men and women, in some societies the latter predominate. All age groups and social classes use the product. Areca nut has a long history of use and is deeply ingrained in many sociocultural and religious activities. An increased risk for the development of oral malignancy in "areca nut only users" is reported. Adding tobacco to the quid is indeed a confounder in many studies, but there are some populations such as Taiwanese who do not add tobacco to the betel and areca quid. The reported relative risk for oral cancer among those who chew areca only in the Taiwanese population is 58.4 (95% confidence interval 7.6 to 447.6). The admixture of tobacco products further increases the likelihood of developing oral malignancy. Both duration and daily frequency of areca use increase the risk of developing cancer, suggesting a dose response relation.

There are many substances, exposure to which can result in head and neck cancer, the elaboration of every substance is beyond the scope of this book. Notably, formaldehyde leads to development of nasopharyngeal carcinoma and was labelled a carcinogen based on this association.

Prior radiation therapy has been implicated in the genesis of many human malignancies, but the relationship with head and neck cancer remains weak. Diet also, has not been found much of a contributory or protective factor. Although consumption of vegetables and fruits seems to confer some protection. Interestingly, nasopharyngeal carcinoma has been found to be associated with preserved meat consumption.

In a study done in North Carolina reduced odds of head and neck cancer were found for the fruit, vegetables, and lean protein dietary pattern (for highest quartile vs. lowest, odds ratio = 0.53). The fried foods, high-fat and processed meats, and sweets pattern was positively associated only with laryngeal cancer (odds ratio = 2.12). These findings underline the importance of a dietary pattern rich in fruits and vegetables and low in high-fat and processed meats and sweets for prevention of head and neck cancer.

Genetic factors underlie every aspect of oncology and head and neck cancers are no exceptions. The role that these factors play doesn't impact the current management strategies. Extrapolating data from lung cancer studies, it is clear that individuals differ in their susceptibility to the carcinogenic effects of tobacco and other carcinogens owing to variations in metabolism, especially the cytochrome mechanism. How this individual susceptibility could translate into clinical practice remains to be explored.

Another very important and often overlooked cause of head and neck cancers is chronic mechanical irritation due to misaligned teeth and ill-fitting dentures. Many studies have been done to evaluate the role of chronic trauma in carcinogenesis. Experimental animal studies have suggested that chronic trauma may result in cancer formation by two mechanisms. It has been proposed that persistent mechanical irritation causes DNA damage and may eventually result in cancer formation. This has been proven by increased activity of poly-ADP-ribose polymerase in cases with chronic trauma.

According to the second proposed mechanism, chronic mucosal trauma results in inflammation, thereby releasing chemical mediators such as cytokine, prostaglandins, and tumor necrosis factor. Such an inflammation leads to oxidative stress. This could induce genetic and epigenetic changes damaging DNA, inhibiting its repair, altering transcription factors, preventing apoptosis, and stimulating angiogenesis, thus resulting in carcinogenesis. In a nutshell, inflammation may act at different steps and result in cancer formation.

A review of 22 articles, which described chronic mucosal trauma as risk factors for oral cancers showed that chronic mucosal irritation resulting from ill-fitting dentures may be considered a risk factor for the development of oral cancer, such cancers occur commonly over the lateral border of the tongue. However, no association has been proven between the duration of denture use and cancer formation. In patients without any addiction, such cancers occur more frequently in females. These cancers may present with an early nodal disease but their prognosis and outcomes have not been studied separately till now.

CHAPTER 2: PRINCIPLES OF PATHOLOGY

Head and neck region can harbour many types of benign and malignant conditions, and due to the heterogeneity of the tissues involved, almost all types of cancers can be encountered, including squamous cell carcinoma, lymphoma, sarcoma, melanoma, basal cell carcinoma et cetera along with many benign conditions as well. The term head and neck cancer denotes the histology "squamous cell carcinoma", unless otherwise specified, as this is the most common histology. In this chapter, we will discuss the principles of pathology in malignancies of head and neck region, as well as benign and premalignant conditions.

The principles of pathology in head and neck cancer pertain mainly to squamous cell carcinoma.

Although cytology is useful in certain situations, most of the times a surgical specimen, biopsy specimen or cell block preparation is required for proper management planning. The squamous cell histology has been further explored and many systems have evolved to further categorise the patients in different subgroups. These features include the grades of differentiation, patterns of infiltration and margin status. Although these features many times prove to be observer dependent, and their inclusion in the TNM staging system and treatment guidelines is not streamlined to a sufficient extent, still they are reported worldwide and aid in clinical decision making.

Procuring a biopsy specimen is obviously the first step in performing pathological examination. Biopsy can be of two basic types, excisional or incisional. Excisional biopsy is done for smaller lesions, and it can provide other useful information besides the histology, like invasion. Incisional biopsy is used for clinically larger lesions in which a sample is obtained using a specialised needle. Surface cytology or aspiration cytology specimens can be obtained in lieu of biopsy but these are seldom performed. Another very popular and frequent practice is to use frozen section specimens, that are obtained at the time of ongoing surgery; although the utility of this practice has not been studied well.

Assessment of margins is undoubtedly very important for treatment decisions, although it remains tricky. The key in proper assessment of margins is the communication between surgeon and pathologist, because what matters is the orientation of the sample obtained by the pathologist, and because the margins exist in two dimensional plane under a microscope while the specimen has a three dimensional orientation, the interpretation is highly dependant upon the proper orientation of the specimen.

The National Comprehensive Cancer Network (NCCN) has formulated a set of guidelines related to margins of resection, and these are used in the recommendations of the College of American Pathologists: Complete resection of the tumor means the "inked" specimen margins are negative for in situ and invasive tumor, adequate margins vary by tumor site, clear margin is defined as at least 5 mm from invasive tumor and close margin is defined as less than 5 mm from invasive tumor.

Premalignant lesions pose a unique challenge. They may herald the onset of malignancy, may remain unchanged over prolonged periods of time and patient anxiety levels often dictate the diagnostic and therapeutic modalities used.

Leukoplakia generally refers to a firmly attached white patch on a mucous membrane which is associated with an increased risk of cancer. The edges of the lesion are typically abrupt and the lesion changes with time. These lesions are asymptomatic but they are premalignant, with a variable (3% to more than 15%) chance of progression to invasive cancer. Generally the causes are the same as those of frank squamous cell carcinoma of head and neck like tobacco, alcohol and betel nut. The biopsy of these lesions is not specific and consistently shows keratin accumulation with or without abnormal cells. These features upon pathological examination are important to denote, as the presence of abnormal cells may warrant surgical or laser removal of these lesions. Otherwise they are merely observed and the patient is strictly advised to abstain from smoking, drinking or any other contributory habits.

Erythroplakia is the presence of erythematous, red colored, patches on mucous membranes. It is a diagnosis of exclusion, and is only made when other causes of such lesions have been exhausted. This term is analogous to leukoplakia, which describes white patches. Together, these are the two traditionally accepted types of premalignant lesion in the mouth, when a lesion contains both red and white areas, the term "speckled leukoplakia" or "erythroleukoplakia" is used. Although oral erythroplakia is much less common than leukoplakia, erythroplakia carries a significantly higher risk of containing dysplasia or carcinoma in situ, and of eventually transforming into invasive squamous cell carcinoma.

Another form of such lesions is simply known as squamous hyperplasia, these are the same as leukoplakia but are not having essentially the predominant white discoloration seen in the latter. The cause of such lesions is chronic irritation most of the times, from sharp teeth or ill fitting dentures, the malignant potential of such lesions is not defined but once they are identified the insulting mechanical factor should be taken care of.

The next kind of premalignant lesion is squamous dysplasia. The normal development of cells lining the structures in head and neck is tightly regulated and follows the rules of cell differentiation. But when the normal pattern is somehow disrupted, dysplasia results. Dysplasia identifies cells that have lost their "polarity", whose nuclear features have become dysmorphic and overall shape and integrity of intercellular connections is lost. World health organisation has developed a tiered system for grading of dysplasia in mild, moderate, severe and carcinoma-in-situ types. This designation depends on the progressive one thirds of epithelium involved, starting from the base, eventually culminating in the involvement of the whole of the epithelium when it's known as carcinoma-in-situ. The grading system is not precise and it's presently not possible to reliably predict behaviour of a particular type of dysplasia. While some high grade dysplasia may spontaneously disappear, the lower grade ones may progress.

Now coming to invasive squamous cell carcinoma, recently there has been some major advancements in our understanding of these cancers. Just a few years back, these were considered a single entity but now there is a clear differentiation between two of its subtypes, namely tobacco related and HPV related. This classification has implications on diagnostic methods, staging and treatment. Tobacco (and alcohol) related squamous cancers have features like inactivation of p53 with peculiar chromosomal abnormalities, but the identification of these is not part of clinical practice and is more of research purposes.

HPV is being increasingly recognised as a cause of squamous cell cancer of head and neck of the lymphoid-rich oropharyngeal region especially in young patients, in whom traditional risk factors are not at play. It inactivates the retinoblastoma gene (Rb), and stops its negative feedback on viral E6 and E7 proteins, which results in overexpression of tumor suppressor protein p16. This protein is now mandatorily assessed in all oropharyngeal tumors. There are many precise tests available for the illustration of the HPV subtype present in such patients but the immunohistochemistry performed on the biopsy specimen is the most practiced and accepted method.

Invasive squamous cell carcinoma is a term designated for the dysplastic/cancerous cells which infiltrate the connective tissue by breaching the basement membrane. The classical model of the development of these types of malignancies emphasizes on the usual progression from dysplasia to carcinoma-in-situ and ultimately leading to invasive squamous cell carcinoma but many times the preexisting carcinoma-in-situ is not identified, and the first presentation is in the form of invasive carcinoma.

Keratinization is the hallmark, it's often present in the form of pearls of keratin within the dysplastic tumor cells. The degree of resemblance of these cancers with the developmental phases of normal squamous epithelium has led to many systems of grading, like well, moderately and poorly differentiated squamous cell carcinoma. Another, maybe more useful, categorisation is keratinising and non-keratinising, tumors of oral cavity belongs to the former and those of oropharynx belong to the latter category.

Other important prognostic information can be obtained by histological examination of the primary site, the most important of which is the depth of invasion and tumor thickness. The depth of invasion parameter has been incorporated in the eighth edition of AJCC, and is a predictor of lymph nodal and systemic metastases. In one study the patients were divided into three groups based on the depth of invasion into those with 1–5 mm, 6–10 mm and > 10 mm. Risk of local recurrence and nodal metastasis were 15% and 23%, 20% and 34%, and 40% and 53% respectively. This study concluded that depth of invasion more than 10 mm is associated with poor outcomes.

Other features like lymphovascular invasion and perineural invasion are also to be determined, as some trials have used these features to decide the treatment planning.

Variants of squamous cell carcinoma

Verrucous carcinoma is a variant of squamous cell carcinoma, comprising only 5% of all varieties. It is slow growing and poses unique challenges in diagnosis. Deep biopsy is a must in such lesions because of the confusing superficial findings that are often encountered. Like conventional squamous cell carcinoma these lesions also exist on a spectrum of relatively benign to invasive subsets.

Overall it's not an aggressive malignancy. Surgery is the primary modality of treatment, with complete excision being the goal although many a times difficult to achieve. Radiation was thought to be detrimental in these cases, as it was feared that radiation would transform this otherwise slow growing malignancy to an aggressive one, but these fears have never been validated and no longer considered legitimate.

Basaloid squamous cell carcinoma is found mostly in association with HPV16 positivity and affects oropharynx. It is characterised by peculiar basaloid cells. This variety shows scant keratinisation, if any. Local metastatic potential is high whereas distant metastasis occur with lower frequency than conventional squamous cell carcinoma.

Spindle cell variant of squamous cell carcinoma is very tricky and sometimes misleading. One fact ought to be clearly understood that it is not a sarcoma. Sarcomas can occur in head and neck region but the mere presence of spindle cells should not be a diagnostic feature. Many times it's hard to differentiate these cells from those of sarcomatous cells, so in most cases immunohistochemistry is to be undertaken, which then will clearly show the true nature of cells. This variant has high local recurrent potential. Some studies have suggested that it can be relatively radioresistant, but this has not been validated and treatment principles remain the same as that of conventional squamous cell carcinoma.

Nasopharyngeal carcinoma arises from the epithelial lining of the nasopharynx. The presentation of these cancers is usually with large cervical lymph nodal masses. The Trotter's syndrome is a cluster of symptoms associated with certain types of advanced nasopharyngeal carcinoma. Symptoms include unilateral conductive deafness due to middle ear effusion, trigeminal neuralgia due to perineural spread, soft palate immobility and difficulty opening mouth. These cancers are associated with Epstein-Barr virus. There are two types of nasopharyngeal carcinoma: keratinising and non-keratinising. Although epidemiology varies but non-keratinising type is more common. Epstein-Barr virus can be demonstrated as a causal agent in many cases using sophisticated tests.

Sinonasal undifferentiated carcinoma (SNUC) is a rare malignancy, it's an aggressive neoplasm that is clinico-pathologically distinct from other poorly differentiated malignancies of the nasal cavity and sinuses. SNUC is believed to originate from schneiderian epithelium or from the nasal ectoderm of the paranasal sinuses. SNUC typically presents as a rapidly enlarging tumor mass involving multiple (sinonasal tract) sites, often with an evidence of extension beyond the anatomic confines of the sinonasal tract.

Given the undifferentiated nature of this malignancy, however, immunohistochemical analysis is extremely helpful. With the use of a panel of markers, positive staining for neuron-specific enolase and chromogranin, cytokeratins 7, 8 and 19, nonreactive to S-100 and non-expression of vimentin. These findings suggest that the tumor is of epithelial origin and lacks any evidence of neuroendocrine, muscle, melanocyte or leukocyte differentiation. This allows proper classification of the tumor as an SNUC - a malignant tumor of the sinus (sinonasal) that is of epithelial origin (carcinoma), but lacks evidence of keratin production (undifferentiated).

Since the initial recognition of SNUC as a distinct clinicopathological entity, treatment regimens have evolved to include the current recommendation of combined radial resection, radiotherapy and chemotherapy. Despite this aggressive therapy, outcome has remained dismal, with the mean survival time being less than a year after diagnosis.

Adenocarcinomas of the sinonasal tract may originate from respiratory surface epithelium or the underlying seromucinous glands. These malignancies are divided into salivary-type adenocarcinomas and non-salivary-type adenocarcinomas. The latter are further divided into intestinal-type and non intestinal-type adenocarcinomas.

Schneiderian papillomas are benign neoplasms that are associated with three key characteristics: tendency to recur, capacity for local destruction, and association with squamous cell carcinoma. These neoplasms arise from a unique area of the respiratory epithelium, termed the schneiderian mucosa. They are classified into inverting, fungiform and oncocytic varieties. The inverting and fungiform varieties are the most common, and the inverting variety has the highest rate of association with malignancy. The inverting and oncocytic varieties are classically found on the lateral nasal wall with extension into the adjacent sinuses. The fungiform lesion is typically found on the nasal septum. Treatment of these lesions is primarily surgical, with rather aggressive surgery mandated in most cases. There may be a limited role for radiation therapy and close follow-up of these patients is mandatory.

Salivary glands in humans can be divided into two broad groups, major and minor. Overall the malignancies arising out of salivary glands are varied in every aspect, from biology to treatment options. They are classified in many ways, commonly the grouping is done on the basis of the cells of origin. It's beyond the scope of this chapter to enumerate and elucidate all the types, so the more common ones will be discussed here.

Pleomorphic adenoma is a benign tumour, arising

most commonly from the parotid gland, although it may arise from any. As its name suggests it has a variety of components. In case the different components can't be identified then the diagnosis is monomorphic adenoma, which is a separate consideration. Although it's a benign condition, it's notorious for local recurrence, especially in cases where adequate margins are not obtained. So in cases of affliction of parotid gland with this neoplasm, the surgical approach should be that of superficial parotidectomy with care taken to preserve the facial nerve. Tumours involving the deep lobe pose difficult surgical problems but principles remain the same.

Sometimes malignant transformation of pleomorphic adenoma takes place, and any sort of histology may arise due to the transformative process, although carcinoma are most common. When such happenstance takes place, it's imperative to abandon conservative approach and radical surgical measures should be taken along with adjuvant treatment depending upon clinical features.

Mucoepidermoid carcinoma is the most common of malignant salivary gland tumours. It has been graded depending upon histologic features, which correlate with survival outcomes. These tumours have high expression of EGFR and low expression of HER2. Mucoepidermoid carcinoma (MEC) is believed to arise from the reserve cells of excretory ducts, and the tumor consists of three cell types: epidermoid cells, mucous cells and poorly differentiated intermediate cells. It is well known that MEC displays a variety of biological behaviors, and that while the high-grade MEC is a highly aggressive tumor, its low-grade counterpart usually demonstrates a more benign nature. Several systems have been proposed to grade this neoplasm, but none has been universally accepted. A recent grading schema (Goode's grading) has been shown to be reproducible and to be predictive of the patient's outcome by defining low, intermediate and high-grade tumors using five histopathologic features. However, some patients with low-grade MECs according to Goode's grading at its early stage have occasionally developed distant metastases. Consequently, different investigators have proposed a variety of sub-classifications and histopathologic grading criteria in order to predict clinical prognosis of MECs more accurately. These tumors have high levels of expression of EGFR and a minority express HER2 but the clinical implications are not well studied.

Adenoid cystic carcinoma is the second most common salivary gland tumor; it's a malignant tumor with a deceptively benign histologic appearance characterized by indolent, locally invasive growth with high propensity for local recurrence and distant metastasis. The tumor is composed of basaloid cells with small, angulated, and hyperchromatic nuclei and scant cytoplasm arranged into three prognostically significant patterns: cribriform, tubular, and solid. Some tumors undergo dedifferentiation into a high-grade form. Numerous studies have attempted to elucidate accurate histologic prognostic features but have often yielded conflicting results. Microarray analysis and gene expression profiling have provided new potential diagnostic and prognostic markers. However, tumor grade, stage, lymph node metastasis, invasion of major nerves, and margin status remain the most consistent predictors of prognosis. The combination of surgery and postoperative radiation therapy has improved locoregional control of the disease. Despite this achievement, late local recurrence and distant metastasis rates remain high and may occur decades after initial diagnosis.

Polymorphous adenocarcinoma was previously considered a type of adenoid cystic carcinoma, but there are subtle differences despite the fact that both of these malignancies invade perineural spaces and have high loco-regional recurrence rates. As a differentiating feature, polymorphous adenocarcinoma of salivary glands doesn't express c-kit whereas adenoid cystic carcinoma may. Surgery is the primary modality of treatment and adjuvant treatment may be needed depending on the pathological features.

Head and neck sarcomas, olfactory neuroblastoma (esthesioneuroblastoma), juvenile nasopharyngeal angiofibromas, ameloblastomas et cetera are rare tumors which we will discuss in subsequent sections dedicated to these neoplasms.

CHAPTER 3: CHEMOPREVENTION

The National Cancer Institute defines chemoprevention as "the use of drugs, vitamins, or other agents to try to reduce the risk of, or delay the development or recurrence of, cancer." The causative agents of head and neck cancer have demonstrable effects on the normal epithelium and related structures. Because the exposure to these agents is chronic and the development of invasive cancer is a multi-step process, there are many opportunities to implement the concept of chemoprevention. It is important to understand that the cancer which ultimately arises is a manifestation of a much larger cancerous change that has been taking place for quite some time and even after the development and successful treatment of the primary cancer, chances remain of the development of another cancer due to the damage incurred to other structures in the whole of upper aerodigestive tract, known as field cancerization.

The most important step in the prevention of development of head and neck cancer is avoidance of further damage by stopping the consumption of tobacco, alcohol or any other inciting factors. That being said, it's logically not enough for the prevention because the damage which has already occurred, persists and can give rise to cancer. Here comes the role of chemoprevention as it can not only reverse the deleterious changes and thus prevent development of cancer in the first place, but also will help in the prevention of cancers that may arise after treatment of a primary cancer. Screening for head and neck cancer can be considered in high risk individuals, but there is a dearth of consensus guidelines and any screening program has associated inherent harms.

Field cancerization is an important phenomenon and should be understood in detail. The concept and the definition of field cancerization was first introduced by Slaughter *et al.* in 1953, when he analyzed the tissues adjacent to squamous cell carcinoma. The concept was first examined in the aerodigestive tract, where multiple primary tumors and local recurrent tumors originate from the anaplastic tendency of multiple cells. The term *lateral cancerization* was coined later to suggest the lateral spread of tumors, which occurs due to a progressive transformation of the tissue adjacent to the tumor rather than the expansion of pre-existing cancer cells into the adjacent tissue. On the basis of a broad analysis of 783 carcinoma patients, Slaughter *et al.* observed that the entire epithelium adjacent to the tumor exhibited more than one independent area of malignancy. Later, the expression of *field cancerization* was adopted, as these findings suggested that the exposure to carcinogen-induced mucosal changes makes the adjacent area susceptible to multiple malignant foci. The concept of field cancerization was extended to other organs, including oropharynx, esophagus, lungs, stomach, colon, cervix, anus, skin and bladder. The oral cavity was proven to be most susceptible to this process, as it is exposed to a wide range of environmental carcinogens which affect the entire mucosa and result into the simultaneous occurrence of premalignant states. This led to various molecular analyses to investigate the genetic mutations and clonality to validate this carcinogenesis model. In particular these findings were reported in 1950's when the Watson and Crick model was first described. Later numerous molecular techniques provided unequivocal evidence supporting the concepts proposed by Slaughter *et al.*

Warren and Gates initially formulated a set of criteria to diagnose multiple primary carcinomas which were modified later by Hong *et al.* The criteria to be met are as follows: i) the neoplasm must be distinct and anatomically separate. A multi-centric primary neoplasm is diagnosed when a dysplastic mucosa is present next to it; ii) a potential second primary carcinoma which represents a metastasis or a local relapse should be excluded. It has to occur *3 years* after the initial diagnosis or it should be separate from the first tumor by at least *2 cm* from the normal epithelium.

Numerous factors determine the progression of a field into a new tumor and must therefore be accurately reviewed and followed up. A premalignant field often requires a much longer period of approximately 67-96 months to progress into an invasive carcinoma.

As is evident from this discussion, this cancerization of the entire upper aerodigestive tract due to the shared etiological agents precludes the definite management of all the potential sites, as it's not possible to reliably assess every site. This is the reason why the survival rates of advanced head and neck cancers are not improving despite proper management of primary site; due to the high rate of recurrence and second malignancies.

Hopes for arresting the development of neoplastic disease arise from research concerning chemoprevention. Chemoprevention implies the application of natural or pharmacological factors, in order to slow down, restrain, or cause regression of the cancerogenic process in people with elevated risk of neoplastic disease. The authors of the concept of neoplasm chemoprevention are L.W. Wattenberg and M.B. Sporn. Their studies made in the 1960s and 1970s provided the basis for further research in that respect. Extending the knowledge concerning the causes of cancerogenesis on molecular level created the basis for trying to find specific chemopreventive agents. Due to the mechanism and stage, at which chemopreventive agents act, they may be divided into blocking (anti-initiative) and suppressive ones. Because some compounds may act both at the stage of initiation and promotion of carcinogenesis, the division that is more often applied is not based on the stage of tumour development, but on the basis of the cascade of events which they interfere with.

One can distinguish three main strategies of chemoprevention: primary, secondary, and tertiary. Primary chemoprevention is addressed to healthy individuals with elevated risk of cancer development, with reference to the population of, e.g., those exposed to carcinogen action, at present or in the past. Examples of primary chemoprevention include HPV vaccination and discontinuation of tobacco smoking. Secondary chemoprevention has the task of inhibiting the progress of existing pre malignancies. Tertiary chemoprevention concerns prevention of second primary tumours (SPTs) as well as recurrence in patients who have gone successfully through the treatment of squamous cell carcinoma lesion.

Some chemical compounds have been tried for application in both chemoprevention and in the treatment of carcinomas. Depending on the fact whether a given chemical substance is used in the treatment of cancer or in its prevention and the type of prevention, the balance of gains and losses resulting from a given intervention change and—what follows—the acceptable adverse effects and permissible toxicity level also vary, as well as the permissible maximum dose resulting from that.

Retinoids constitute a group of chemical compounds comprising vitamin A, the natural analogs of vitamin A, and its synthetic derivatives. Retinoids bind with specific nuclear receptors: RAR (retinoid acid receptor) and RXR (retinoid X receptor), which perform the function of transcriptive factors. After binding the retinoid with the receptor, the RARE (retinoid acid response element) sequences may be launched, which are present in promoter areas, as well as RXRE (retinoid X response element), which are adjacent to some 100 genes and may influence their expression. This mechanism controls the development and differentiation of both regular and neoplastic cells. Retinoids inhibit the expression of transcriptive factor AP-1 (activator protein 1), enhance the expression of TGF-β2 (transforming growth factor β2), modulate histone acetylation, and may induce apoptosis.

The first studies concerning chemoprevention focused upon attempts of reversing the premalignancy lesions in the mouth cavity (mainly leukoplakia and submucous fibrosis) as those lesions may easily be subject to biopsy and observation of the clinical condition. The efficiency of treating leukoplakia with 13-cis-retinoic acid (isotretinoin) has been demonstrated and proven by Hong. The compound was administered in the doses of 1-2 mg/kg of body mass/day, for 3 months, which resulted in reduction of the size of leukoplakia foci in 67% of subjects and regression of dysplasia in 54% of patients. Sankaranarayanan et al. examined 160 subjects, who have been divided into 3 groups. For 12 months, the first group was administered vitamin A in the doses of 300 000 IU/ week, the second received β-carotene in the doses of 360 mg/week, and the third was administered placebo. Promising results were obtained, particularly in the group receiving vitamin A (lesions subsided in 52% of subjects from group one, 33% of subjects from group two, and 10% from the group receiving placebo). Those promising results provided the basis for studies concerning the application of retinoids in tertiary prevention that is prevention of SPTs occurrence and recurrence of the disease in patients who successfully completed squamous cell carcinoma treatment.

Many studies ensued following these initial studies and the findings have been equivocal. While the ideal dosing regimen is not known, many times the use of retinoids is incorporated in clinical planning. That being said, it's important to note that retinoids are not devoid of adverse effects and the usage should also take into consideration the coexisting health conditions of the patients and pregnancy.

In head and neck carcinomas, increased production of prostaglandins has been detected, particularly of prostaglandin E2 (PGE2), in comparison with healthy tissue. Cyclooxygenase (COX) catalyzes the first stage of transformation of arachidonic acid, common for the pathway of prostaglandin, prostacyclin, and thromboxane synthesis. In the second pathway of arachidonic acid metabolism, initiated by lipoxygenases, leukotrienes are formed. Cyclooxygenase is present in two main isoenzymes, COX-1 and COX-2. COX-1 is an enzyme which is constitutively synthesized. COX-2, on the other hand, is an enzyme whose synthesis is induced by proinflammatory cytokines and growth factors, which increase its synthesis in tissues in case of inflammatory condition or neoplasm. In most healthy tissues this enzyme is not detected. Increased activity of this enzyme has been confirmed, among other things, in head and neck squamous cell carcinomas, as well as in dysplastic lesions in that area. Prostaglandins synthesized by COX-2 stimulate the proliferation of cells, act as immunosuppressants (which minimize the chances of the immune system to destroy irregular cells), as well as promote angiogenesis and metastasis. Increased synthesis of PGE2, referred to above, results in reduced frequency of apoptosis. In connection with that, COX inhibitors started to be studied as chemopreventive factors.

Non Steroidal anti-inflammatory drugs (NSAIDs) inhibit both isoenzymes, which is demonstrated by adverse effect, among others, on the alimentary tract mucosa, thus promoting the development of gastric ulcers and in some cases causing bleeding from the ulcers. For that reason, selective inhibitors of COX-2 have been introduced to the market, as anti-inflammatory drugs deprived of that adverse effect. Celecoxib was one of the first such compounds. The research concerning its application as a chemopreventive agent in head and neck squamous cell carcinomas resulted in contradictory conclusions, what is more, the studies were conducted on relatively small groups. In the study conducted on 22 patients with pre malignancies in the mouth cavity, the level of PGE2 was monitored, as well as its changes in response to the administered celecoxib. Biopsies of the morbid tissues were performed: the first one after 12 weeks of treatment, and another one after 12 months of drug administration. Reduced level of PGE2 was noted, as well as less dysplasia. In the randomized phase 2 study, with 50 subjects, the first group of patients received celecoxib in the doses of 100 mg, twice a day; in the second group the drug dose was 200 mg, also administered twice daily; the third group received placebo. Like in the previous study, the subjects had confirmed pre malignancies of the mucous membranes in the oral cavity. Unfortunately, after 12 weeks of the study, no advantageous, chemopreventive action was observed in study subjects. In order to eliminate the possible adverse effects, also a topical application of the drug was tested, which may be applied for a longer time, without risk for the cardiovascular system. In the randomized study, flushing of the mouth cavity with selective inhibitor of COX-2 (ketorolac) was applied. The number of study subjects was 57; they flushed the oral cavity with 10 ml of 0.1% solution of ketorolac twice a day, for 30 seconds each time. Unfortunately, no statistically significant differences were noted between the group receiving placebo and the group administered the drug.

Epidermal growth factor receptor (EGFR) is a protein belonging to the family of receptors of ErbB, which is present on the cell surface. EGFR is composed of an extracellular domain, which binds with the receptor ligand, transmembrane domain, and intracellular domain having tyrosine kinase activity. The ligands for the receptor are proteins from the growth factor family, which have a domain of structure homological to the epidermal growth factor (EGF). After connecting the ligand to receptor, a cell activation cascade is launched, which may contribute to transformation into a cell with potentially malicious phenotype, in case of excessive activity of the receptor. EGFR overexpression was confirmed in numerous types of neoplasms, also in more than 80% of HNSCC. This resulted in searching for agents that block the activity of EGFR, which would have a two-way action: creation of antibodies that block the receptor and development of low molecular weight inhibitors of tyrosine kinase (TKIs).

The cetuximab monoclonal antibody found application for adjunctive treatment during radiotherapy in advanced forms of head and neck squamous cell carcinomas improving 5-year survival. In a study of Bonner et al. 5-year overall survival was 45.6% among patients receiving radiotherapy and cetuximab, whereas only 36.4% in the group treated with radiotherapy alone. The results of adding cetuximab to chemotherapy consisting of cisplatin or carboplatin combined with 5-fluorouracil are not so good. Cetuximab (Erbitux) also significantly increased the medium overall survival and the medium progression-free period. However, the median overall survival was still short, 10.1 months in the cetuximab group compared to 7.4 months in patients receiving chemotherapy alone. These results come from the randomized phase III study EXTREME (Erbitux in First-Line Treatment of Recurrent or Metastatic Head and Neck Cancer) and indicate that statistical significance of differences in overall survival observed in this study may not always mean clinical significance as statistically better overall survival was still clinically poor. Administered in monotherapy (for patients with cancer resistant to chemotherapy), cetuximab provided response in 13% of treated individuals. A somewhat lower efficacy was demonstrated by the following two antibodies: panitumumab and zalutumumab. Panitumumab was administered to a large group of patients, in combination with chemotherapy (SPECTRUM study), while zalutumumab was tested on the group of patients with neoplasms resistant to chemotherapy. In both cases, prolonged progression-free survival (PFS) was achieved. Those results provided the basis for applying the EGR receptor inhibitors in studies concerning chemoprevention in HNSCC. In the studies performed on oral cavity carcinogenesis model, induced in mice by 4NQO (4-Nitroquinoline-1-oxide) carcinogen dissolved in water, a substantial reduction (69%) was demonstrated, of both dysplasia and squamous cell carcinoma by means of erlotinib, a low molecular weight inhibitor of tyrosine kinase domain of EGF receptor.

Unfortunately, such good results did not get repeated in the study performed on cetuximab application in humans, the EPOC study (Erlotinib Prevention of Oral Cancer). The patients that qualified for participating in the study belonged to a high risk group, as regards the development of squamous cell carcinoma, due to advanced dysplasia, confirmed loss of heterozygosity (LOH), a potential risk marker of pre malignancies turning malignant, in one of the typical locations for head and neck cancerogenesis, or due to the history of head and neck carcinoma. A group of 150 patients with confirmed loss of heterozygosity qualified for the study, they were administered erlotinib in the doses of 150 mg/day, for 12 months, and were followed-up for another two years. The disease free survival (DFS) did not change, what is more, in about half of the subjects the erlotinib doses were reduced, due to adverse effects. Much hope arises from the results of the study concerning vandetanib, conducted on animal model of carcinogenesis (4-NQO). Vandetanib is an inhibitor of two receptors: for Vascular Endothelial Growth Factor (VEGF), and for Epithelial Growth Factor (EGF). The application of vandetanib for 24 weeks in mice was linked with significant reduction of the percentage of dysplasia or cancer occurrence (from 96% in the placebo group to 28% in the group receiving the drug). Phase I studies were conducted, concerning the application of erlotinib as a chemopreventive agent in 12 patients diagnosed with advanced premalignancies, mainly leukoplakia, dysplasia of low, medium, and high degree, as well as cancer in situ. The therapy lasted for about 5 months and comprised combined oral application of erlotinib, in the doses 50, 75, and 100 mg as escalating dose, and oral administration of celecoxib, in the dose of 400 mg, 2 times a day for 6 months. The control was performed by means of biopsy after 3, 6, and 12 months. In 43% of patients the histological picture of lesions improved, while in 29% no further deterioration was noted. Also, reduced activity of EGF and p-ERK receptor was observed, which is one of the proteins of the MAPK/ERK signaling pathways, launched as a result of EGFR stimulation. Those results are a promising prognostic sign for further studies. The limitations of erlotinib doses were related to rash being an adverse effect.

Reduction of the amount of folic acid influences the lack of balance in the synthesis of uracil and thymine, pyrimidine bases that form RNA and DNA, which—in turn—causes disturbances in DNA synthesis and its repair. What is more, deficiency of folic acid contributes to problems with DNA methylation and difficulties with control and expression of proto oncogenes.

DR. BHRATRI BHUSHAN

Folic acid deficiency is connected with increased exposure to neoplasm occurrence. A research was conducted on 745 patients with cancer of the oral cavity and pharynx, who responded to a questionnaire concerning eating habits, with particular attention paid to the consumption of food containing folic acid. The results obtained were compared with results from the control group of 1772 subjects who were hospitalized due to other ailments, not connected with neoplasia. It was concluded that the consumption of folic acid in the diet, in medium or big amounts, may prevent the occurrence of neoplastic lesions in the mouth cavity, even in case of alcohol abuse, alcohol being an agent which fosters the formation of neoplasms.

Vitamin E is a group of chemical compounds soluble in organic fats, which includes tocopherols and tocotrienols. Tocotrienols are unoxidized forms of vitamin E, which demonstrate antioxidative activity. Vitamin E not only protects cells from oxidants, but also takes part in provision of nutrients to cells, strengthens blood vessel walls, and protects red blood cells from premature decomposition. For humans, the most vital role is that performed by α-tocopherol, the most biologically active form of vitamin E which, similar to retinoids, was the subject of many studies concerning chemoprevention. A randomized study conducted by Bairati et al., focused on the influence of supplementation with antioxidants soluble in fats, α-tocopherol and β-carotene, upon the occurrence of second primary tumours in patients with HNSCC stage I or II, undergoing radiotherapy. The plan was to administer both antioxidants during radiotherapy and for the following 3 years. During the study, administration of β-carotene was discontinued, whereas the supplementation with α-tocopherol was maintained. This was caused by ethical reasons, resulting from the report that emerged at that time, concerning increased incidence of lung cancer during supplementation with β-carotene. In patients receiving large doses of α-tocopherol (400 IU/d) increased mortality was observed, with reference to the group which did not get the supplementation. When mentioning that study, one should keep in mind the fact that one of the mechanisms behind the therapeutic effects of radiotherapy in the treatment of neoplasms is the generation of reactive forms of oxygen, via ionizing radiation, which damage tumour cells. Thus, the negative effects of vitamin E application may be caused by combining its supplementation with radiotherapy.

Yet another interesting attempt at chemoprevention of HNSCC was the development of modified adenovirus ONYX-15, which replicates selectively only in cells with mutated gene p53, destroying them. As mutations of gene p53 occur in some 40-50% cases of HNSCC and in some 45% of dysplastic lesions, the idea was born to apply adenovirus ONYX-15 in patients with dysplasia of the oral cavity. Resolution of dysplasia was observed in 7 of the 19 patients who completed the study. Despite the fact that this kind of treatment was well tolerated, the achieved percentage of positive response to treatment, and the transient nature of the improvement demand much caution in assaying the method.

Many other agents have also been studied regarding chemoprevention for example, mTOR inhibitors, PPARs, curcumin, green tea extract, resveratrol, interferon-alpha etc. No clear cut evidence emerged from these studies, as the studies were not devoid of beneficial effects but those effects didn't amount to a degree sufficient for recommending the unequivocal use of these substances. These and other substances are often used in one context or another but special care should be taken regarding avoidance of situations in which their use may induce harm, like the use of antioxidants during radiation therapy.

The better our understanding of carcinogenesis mechanisms and premalignant lesions biology, the more urgent the finding of suitable clinical, histological, molecular, or genetic markers, which will allow for individually targeted chemoprevention, thus enhancing its efficacy. Also, further studies are needed to find markers, which will allow taking decisions concerning termination or further continuation of chemoprevention.

CHAPTER 4: SCREENING

"Cancer is curable, if detected early" is the holy grail of cancer medicine. No matter how far technology progresses, timely detection will always be the key, be it head and cancer, any other cancer or any disease for that matter. The concept of screening falls in the broader "secondary prevention", which is the next best thing to primary prevention, a few strategies of which were discussed in the previous section.

The problem with head and neck cancer screening is the paucity of long term randomised controlled trial data and the lack of resources for implementation of certain high end practices, especially in the developing world. The advancements recently achieved in endoscopy and in quantitative analysis of hypocellular specimens open new perspectives for secondary prevention. Chromoendoscopy and narrow band imaging (NBI) pinpoint suspicious lesions more easily, confocal endomicroscopy and optical coherence tomography obtain optical sections through those lesions, and hyperspectral imaging classifies lesions according to characteristic spectral signatures. These techniques therefore obtain optical biopsies. Once a "conventional" biopsy has been taken, the plethora of parameters that can be quantified objectively has been increased and could be the basis for an objective and quantitative classification of epithelial lesions (multiparametric cytometry, quantitative histology). Finally, cytomics and proteomics approaches, and lab-on-the-chip technology might help to identify patients at high-risk. The problem with these newer modalities is that they are not validated and the population based sensitivity and specificity are unknown, so care is imperative in implementation even on an individual basis as false positive results or the occasional "overdiagnosis" will call for unnecessary and potentially harmful interventions.

The ultimate aim of any screening program is to identify patients when their cancers are at the earliest stages and most amenable to cure. But this simple goal proves to be elusive due to myriads of factors that come in its way. Resource allotment is one key factor that determines the success or failure and even the wide scale implementation of a screening program. Studies suggest that half of head and neck cancers can either be prevented or can be detected at stages when they can be completely cured. So, a collective effort is needed both by the scientific community and policy making bodies of the government.

Popular belief that preventive and screening measures are always safe and should be pursued rather than the therapeutic strategies once the disease develops, is not true to a large extent; the fact that only breast cancer screening program has been a stellar success among so many other failed or not very beneficial programs, attests to this theory. Screening programs in general are ridden with many pitfalls like false positives, overdiagnosis and, the very problematic, false-negative cases, such called interval-carcinoma which go undetected for a long time since they were non-pathological at screening. For head and neck cancers these hurdles become even more pronounced and the principle reason is the lack of consensus on the identification and subsequent classification of head and neck premalignant lesions and the appropriate strategies to be undertaken once such doubtful lesions are revealed on the screening studies. And the often "decisive" element in such discussions, especially on the front of governmental aid, is the cost-benefit ratio and most of the screening tests fall far behind in the fulfillment of this particular criteria.

The ultimate aim of any screening test is reduction in mortality rates associated with the malignancy being screened. While most of the developed countries lack the resources needed for implementation of most screening programs, the proposition simply seems unrealistic in case of developing countries. When discussing screening programs, the often overlooked aspect by the scientific community is the cost of healthcare that poses an increasing burden on the taxpayer and potential collapse of the healthcare system.

Up to 30% of cancer is estimated to be associated with avoidable risk factors (smoking, alcohol, occupational toxics, but also obesity, loss of mobility); nevertheless, so far the positive influence of a "healthy" lifestyle on cardiovascular disease, colon and breast cancer could not be proven. Substitution with specific nutritients which seem to be sensible at first sight turned out to be devastating on a closer look: addition of calcium and vitamin D did not reduce the number of fractures but instead increase the number of nephroliths, and the "preventive" addition of estrogens and gestagens in postmenopausal women lead to significant additional health problems and massive health costs. This underlines the necessary thorough evaluation of any screening program to prove that there is a positive overall cost-risk-ratio. The evidence must be clearly and objectively documented, and there must not be a negative consequence for not attending a program.

There is a clear paradox between other screening program and head and neck cancer screening. Studies done on reasonably executable head and neck cancer screening strategies, particularly "opportunistic screening", have shown notoriously low compliance rates on part of patients, especially those at high risk. The often accepted tests are a mere physical examination, which may be combined with cytology and endoscopy; but the execution remains far from simple.

The first step in successful formulation and subsequent implementation of a screening program is identification of risk factors and assignment of risk categories to otherwise healthy people.

As we have already discussed, tobacco smoking is a known risk factor for head and neck cancer.

The Heidelberger case-control-study showed that >30 pack years increase the risk for head and neck cancer by the factor 4.8, and >60 pack years by the factor 23.4. It is hard to draw universally applicable parameters, as the studies in this regard in head and neck cancer are clearly lacking, but extrapolation can be contemplated of the studies done in lung cancer and a 30 pack-year smoking history maybe taken as a criteria to select people for screening measures, at least those involving higher priced investigations.

Alcohol is another known risk factor for head and neck cancer. The odds ratio ranges from 9.4 for 75 g ethanol per day and 11.7 for >100 g ethanol per day. In females a consumption of >30 g ethanol per day increases the relative risk for head and neck cancer to 29. Finally, the combination of both, smoking and drinking, has the highest propagating effect on head and neck cancer. This effect is over-additive and dose dependent. The combined consumption of >75 g ethanol per day and >30 pack years increase the odds ratio to 92.

Various occupational poisons have been studied and showed the relative risk to develop head and neck cancer associated with them: asbestos 8.7, cement 12.9, tar 6.6, and dyes/paints/solvents around 3; wood dust is associated with sinonasal adenocarcinoma but it's important to keep in mind that the true effect of these toxins is dependent on duration of exposure and risk varies for different anatomical sites. The combination of smoking and drinking alcohol, along with the aforementioned occupational toxin increases the carcinogenic effect.

Trends are changing in many western countries and more cases of head and neck cancers are being diagnosed in never smokers and never drinkers, partly reflecting the declining prevalence of smokers but also highlighting other factors that were hitherto not paid much attention. These patients generally tend to be younger and females show an increased predilection. Over the time many studies have been done and several risk factors have been identified: >50% were serological positive for HPV16, 45% were passive smokers, 24% had occupational toxics in their history, and 30% had gastroesophageal reflux. Herpes simplex virus and human immunodeficiency virus may also have a role, albeit controversial.

zur Hausen is Nobel laureate for having established the concept of viral etiology in development of cervical cancer. Increasingly, head and neck cancer patients demonstrate presence of human papilloma virus as well. A metaanalysis of 60 publications showed the prevalence for HPV-infection to be 25.9% for all head and neck cancer, highest in oropharynx (35.6%) and larynx (24.0%) and oral cavity cancer (23.5%). In oropharynx in 87% of positive cases were HPV16, whereas in hypopharynx and larynx a higher proportion of HPV18 is seen (17% vs. 38%). This is the basis for the discussion about vaccinating young males against HPV, too.

The knowledge which is vital for any screening program is the origins of the cancer in question and the "steps" that it goes through to ultimately become manifest. The concept of precursor lesion has been proposed for many cancers, and the hypothesis behind it is that any cancer doesn't just spontaneously arise one day, there must be stepwise progression from normal to cancerous tissue. The WHO just states: "Precursor lesions are defined as altered epithelium with a high likelihood to develop into cancer". Clinically in general leukoplakia, erythroplakia, and chronic inflammation are seen, histologically represented as dysplasia and atypia. The problem with this terminology is the lack of standardisation; while in theory it all seems to make sense but practical application is not so simple. And while this stepwise progression model is true to some extent, it is well known that cancer may arise directly from lower grade lesions or even from apparently healthy mucosa. The newer techniques of elucidation of genetic alterations are promising but far from perfect, cumbersome and not validated.

Leukoplakia and erythroplakia on the other hand are clinical diagnosis and seem reproducible among experts. We have already discussed their characteristics in the previous chapter.

So, to summarise, presently the best way to asses premalignant lesions is the proper histopathological examination of a biopsy specimen. It is important to stress here that this technique is very subjective, as put nicely by Lessells et al.: "Histopathological diagnosis is not carried out in an algorithmic process. Individual pathologists have a highly trained visual cortex, such that within a few seconds of looking at a slide a number of conclusions have been drawn and a diagnosis (at least provisional) made. Obviously, individual pathologists are programmed in slightly different ways, accounting for the individual variation seen in a linear spectrum of abnormality such as dysplasia. Even if strict criteria were applied, it is unlikely that any improvement would be more than marginal"

Early detection of head and neck cancers is not a single topic, it has to be broken down into its various anatomical sites to make sense of it all. As some sites, like oral tongue, are easily accessible; whereas sites like hypopharynx are not so much. Obtaining sample also varies greatly in difficulty and the cost of techniques used, so lumping all head and neck cancers is not feasible. Now we shall discuss the most commonly employed methods for screening for common anatomical sites of head and neck.

Oral cavity and oropharynx are not only the commonest sites of development of head and neck cancers in many parts of the world, they are the most easily accessible as well. High quality data is lacking, and often overlooked aspect is cost effectiveness, which as we have already discussed is the main driving factor of a screening program.

One study from India studied the impact of visual inspection on detection and mortality prevention in this context. Of the 13 clusters chosen for the study, seven were randomised to three rounds of oral visual inspection by trained health workers at 3-year intervals and six to a control group during 1996–2004, in Trivandrum district, Kerala, India. Healthy participants aged 35 years and older were eligible for the study. Screen-positive people were referred for clinical examination by doctors, biopsy, and treatment. Outcome measures were survival, case fatality, and oral cancer mortality. Oral cancer mortality in the study groups was analysed and compared by the use of cluster analysis. Analysis was by intention to treat.

Of the 96517 eligible participants in the intervention group, 87655 (91%) were screened at least once, 53312 (55%) twice, and 29102 (30%) three times. Of the 5145 individuals who screened positive, 3218 (63%) complied with referral. 95356 eligible participants in the control group received standard care. 205 oral cancer cases and 77 oral cancer deaths were recorded in the intervention group compared with 158 cases and 87 deaths in the control group (mortality rate ratio 0·79 [95% CI 0·51–1·22]). 70 oral cancer deaths took place in users of tobacco or alcohol, or both, in the intervention group, compared with 85 in controls (0·66 [0·45–0·95]). The mortality rate ratio was 0·57 (0·35–0·93) in male tobacco or alcohol users and 0·78 (0·43–1·42) in female users. This study concluded that oral visual screening can reduce mortality in high-risk individuals and a speculation that it has the potential of preventing at least 37000 oral cancer deaths worldwide.

Coming to other methods that have been studied, it has been hypothesized that abnormal and dysplastic mucosa stains differently than normal mucosa. This led to the development of chromogen assisted visual inspection. In this method the sample is stained with dyes such as toluidine blue or Bengal Rose, and compared with healthy controls of normal mucosa. The application of this method has the principal shortcoming of being overtly observer dependent.

Autofluorescence can aid in the detection of abnormal cells by their virtue of behaving differently to certain light frequencies, it can be modified by applying 5-aminolevulinic acid (5-ALA) topically or systemically. While altered mucosa shows a loss of autofluorescence, it exhibits a gain of 5-ALA-induced fluorescence. For this technique, a sensitivity of 99% and a specificity of 60% are quoted.

Molecular markers like loss of heterozygosity of certain chromosomes have been reproduced many times but the exorbitant costs are prohibitive and so is the lack of validation. Another important and promising marker is detection of HPV16 in healthy individuals using high throughput methods. Recently done studies on this subject give hope for integration of this practice in screening programs, at least in high risk populations.

Classical screening for laryngeal cancer is based on the subjective analysis of conventional indirect laryngoscopy with or without magnification. This can be further enhanced by chromogen assisted analysis and autofluorescence, although studies done exploring the latter aspect have not been fruitful.

Hypopharyngeal cancers may be detected with the help of endoscopy, the pertinent issue being cost of this procedure and the manpower required. Although the survival outcomes can be affected dramatically by the stage at which these cancers are detected.

For the rare primaries like salivary glands, nasopharynx et cetera the screening methods have not been validated in large studies, thus no comments can be made on the appropriate techniques.

Screening is also part of surveillance for second primaries that may develop after treatment of the primary malignancy. We have already discussed the criteria for second primary neoplasms (vide supra). The rate of second primaries ranges from 9 to 19%; 41–46% are synchronous and 54–59% are metachronous. Using panendoscopy up to 85% of synchronous and 67% of metachronous secondary primaries can be detected. In general, a second primary is correlated with a poor survival: the median survival is approximately 25 months.

Repeated endoscopy both, as rigid or as flexible are a standard that can be offered to patients with head and neck cancer and esophageal cancer. The survival time was significantly increased in patients who underwent routine endoscopies as compared to patients with disease-triggered endoscopies from 32 months to 58 months.

PET-CT scans have become an integral part of staging of many cancers, any they have the potential to diagnose synchronous as well as metachronous malignancies in cases of head and neck cancers. But care must be taken of the high radiation dose that is inherent to these scans and the notorious false positive results that lead the diagnostic and therapeutic decision making astray. A study compared PET, PET-CT, CT, and MR and showed that PET-CT had a better accuracy than CT/MR in detecting primaries and metastases (98% vs. 86% and 92% vs. 85%, respectively) but still there were false-positive and false-negative results.

Newer techniques like chromoendoscopy, proteomics, genomic markers et cetera are in development and are bound to face the same problems of balancing sensitivity and specificity in the face of Bayesian principles and more importantly, cost effectiveness and risk-benefit ratio.

To summarize, as proposed by Gogarty et al: "Current levels of public awareness regarding head and neck cancers are suboptimal, despite increased incidence and mortality. Scheduled and opportunistic screening, coupled with efforts to enhance education and health behaviour modification, are highly recommended for pre-defined, high-risk, targeted populations. This can enable early detection and therefore improve morbidity and mortality."

CHAPTER 5: PRINCIPLES OF DIAGNOSIS AND STAGING

The subject of diagnosis and staging of head and neck cancers is complex and vast and in itself a subject of whole another book. This chapter will try to summarize the thought process involved in these exercises and lay a foundation of guideline driven execution of the same. As pointed out at the beginning of this book, for the sake of formulation of guidelines based on disease biology, to standardize the management planning and to accommodate epidemiological data in treatment decision making; head and neck region is divided into the following major subsites:

The oral cavity includes the mucosa of the lips (not the external, dry lips), the buccal mucosa, the anterior tongue, the floor of the mouth, the hard palate, and the upper and lower gingiva. The anterior border of the oral cavity is defined by the portion of the lip that contacts the opposed lip (wet mucosa). The posterior border is defined by the circumvallate papillae of the tongue, the anterior tonsillar pillars (palatoglossus muscles), and the posterior margin of the hard palate. The hard palate defines the superior boundary of the oral cavity. Inferiorly, the oral cavity is defined by the mylohyoid muscles. The lateral boundary of the oral cavity is defined by the buccomasseteric region (buccal mucosa of the cheeks) and the retromolar trigone (which is located behind the mandibular third molar).

The pharynx is divided into the nasopharynx, oropharynx, and hypopharynx. The nasopharynx forms the continuation of the nasal cavity. The boundary between the nasal cavity and nasopharynx is defined by the posterior choanae of the nasal cavity. The nasopharynx is defined superiorly by the basisphenoid and basiocciput (clivus) and inferiorly by the hard and soft palate. The prevertebral muscle and anterior margin of the cervical spine at C1 and C2 levels form the posterior margin of the nasopharynx. The posterolateral boundary of the nasopharynx includes several important structures. The lateral wall of the nasopharynx is elevated by the torus tubarius, a cartilaginous structure that constitutes the opening of the Eustachian tube.

The Eustachian tube allows communication between the middle ear and the nasopharynx through a defect (sinus of Morgagni) of the pharyngobasilar fascia, which lines the nasopharynx. The sinus of Morgagni may allow nasopharyngeal cancer to gain access into the skull base. The fossa of Rosenmüller (lateral nasopharyngeal recess), a common site of nasopharyngeal cancer, is located posterior to the torus tubarius. The nasopharynx also includes the adenoids (nasopharyngeal tonsils), located in the midline roof of the nasopharynx.

The soft palate defines the boundary between the nasopharynx and oropharynx. The oropharynx is separated anteriorly from the oral cavity by the circumvallate papillae and the anterior tonsillar pillars. The palatine tonsils, posterior tonsillar pillars, tongue base (posterior one-third of the tongue), valleculae, soft palate and the posterior pharyngeal wall are structures of the oropharynx. Inferiorly, the oropharynx is defined by the hyoid and the pharyngoepiglottic folds.

The hypopharynx includes the pyriform sinuses, the posterior surface of the larynx (postcricoid area), and the inferior, posterior, and lateral pharyngeal walls.

The larynx, which is divided into three anatomic regions: the supraglottic region, the glottic larynx (true vocal cords and mucosa of the anterior and posterior commissures), and the subglottic larynx, which extends to the inferior border of the cricoid cartilage. The nasal cavity and the paranasal sinuses (maxillary, ethmoid, sphenoid, and frontal).

The major (parotid, submandibular, and sublingual) and minor salivary glands. Minor salivary glands are found within the submucosa throughout the oral cavity, palate, paranasal sinuses, pharynx, larynx, trachea and bronchi, but are most concentrated in the buccal, labial, palatal, and lingual regions.

As can be inferred from the above mentioned facts, the symptomatology of head and neck cancers can encompass a large variety of radically different presentations; while most of the symptoms are reasonably straightforward in their clinical context, many may mislead and throw the clinician off the trail.

People with head and neck cancer often experience the following symptoms or signs. Sometimes, people with head and neck cancer do not have any of these changes. Or, the cause of a symptom may be a different medical condition that is not cancer. Many of these symptoms are site specific but there are exceptions.

- Swelling, a sore or an ulcer that does not heal is the most common symptom

- Red or white patch in the mouth (erythroplakia or leukoplakia)
- Lump, bump, or mass in the head or neck area, with or without pain
- Persistent sore throat
- Foul mouth odor not explained by hygiene
- Hoarseness or change in voice
- Nasal obstruction or persistent nasal congestion
- Frequent nose bleeds and/or unusual nasal discharge
- Difficulty breathing
- Double vision
- Numbness or weakness of a body part in the head and neck region
- Pain or difficulty chewing, swallowing, or moving the jaw or tongue
- Jaw pain
- Blood in the saliva or phlegm, which is mucus discharged into the mouth from respiratory passages
- Loosening of teeth
- Dentures that no longer fit
- Unexplained weight loss
- Fatigue
- Ear pain or infection, which is a "red-flag sign" when it is of the referred type

As discussed in the chapter "principles of pathology", the overwhelming majority of head and neck cancers are squamous cell carcinoma, but many other histologies can also be found in this region, the discussion of staging of which is not the scope of this chapter. The tumor, node, metastases (TNM) staging system of the American Joint Committee on Cancer (AJCC) and the Union for International Cancer Control (UICC) is used to classify cancers of the head and neck. The T classifications indicate the extent of the primary tumor and are site specific, thus being inherently dependent on the anatomy of the primary and the surroundings; on the other hand the N (lymph node) classification is commonly shared among many sites, with a few exceptions.

It all begins with history taking, which not only includes present complaints but also personal habits, family history and history of comorbidities among others, that can help in therapeutic decision making. Physical examination is the next step, the most important concept being inspection and palpation of the assessable structures of head and neck region, which are mostly confined to the oral cavity. Then mirror examination (indirect laryngoscopy) or direct flexible laryngoscopy (fiber optic) are done, not only to visualise the suspected primary site in detail and to obtain biopsy but also to examine potential synchronous malignancies of the upper aerodigestive tract. Ear and nose examination by scopes should also be a part of routine evaluation.

There are two major sites of spread of head and neck cancers: lymph nodes in the cervical region and the lungs. So metastatic work-up is directed to these sites, especially the former. The percentage of occult lymph node metastasis varies between different primary sites, like in the case of carcinoma of tongue the rates are staggering and in cases of hard palate carcinoma cervical lymph node mets are more rare.

The next step is an examination under anesthesia, which is an important, if not the most important part of diagnostic assessment. It helps not only in the delineation of the characteristics of the primary lesion but also procuring of the biopsy specimens. Symptom-directed panendoscopy (laryngoscopy, bronchoscopy and esophagoscopy) reveals a 2.4 to 4.5 percent incidence of second primary tumors of the upper aerodigestive tract, but not of the lower airways. It can be contemplated in heavy smokers and alcohol abusers as a routine test.

In clinical practice imaging studies are often utilized. While they do add information but should not be considered a replacement of the above mentioned clinical examination methods. Techniques like integrated PET-CT scans have shown promise in staging of primary and metastatic sites, but false negatives and false positives are there.

In practice, if a patient presents with enlargement of neck nodes, fine needle aspiration of the node is almost always done to establish a diagnosis of malignancy while other tests are being considered. It's a relatively fast and less morbid procedure which has high sensitivity and specificity and a diagnostic accuracy that ranges from 89 to 98 percent. Sometimes aspirate specimen come back negative, in which case they should be repeated before moving on to perform a core needle or excisional biopsy. Many studies have evaluated the role of doing ultrasound imaging of the neck to detect occult lymph node enlargement, which are not detectable by clinical examination and performing fine needle aspiration of those, results have been mixed but as it's a relatively harmless procedure, it can be integrated in clinical practice.

Imaging studies are important for many reasons, they not only help evaluate the primary site and neck nodes but also distant sites which are not accessible by a physical examination alone.

CT scans are most frequently used modality. There are several advantages of CT scans, like faster acquisition and fine resolution. The tumors show increased enhancement compared to most of the other surrounding structures. Modern CT scanning technology allows for evaluation with 1 mm precision, but 3 mm precision may suffice; although most definitely a resolution poorer than 5 mm is suboptimal.

CT scans are good at looking for soft tissue and bone invasion by the primary tumor. Neck node evaluation, on the other hand, poses some problems, the foremost of which is the size criteria. Expert opinion varies, but mostly the criteria of the minimal axial diameter being more than 10 mm is followed. CT scans can't differentiate between malignant and reactive lymphadenopathy with reliable accuracy.

Disadvantages of CT include radiation exposure, poorer soft tissue contrast compared to MRI, the need to inject iodinated contrast medium to improve contrast with the risk of contrast induced nephropathy and artefacts due to dental amalgam or orthopaedic material, if present. Contraindications to CT can be absolute or relative and include allergy to contrast media, kidney failure with some remaining function, hyperthyroidism, thyroid cancer, bodyweight above 200 kg and inability to lie down. Children are preferentially scanned with MRI or ultrasound when feasible to avoid radiation exposure.

Magnetic resonance imaging (MRI) is an excellent tool for studying soft tissue in detail, with a severe drawback of lack of detailing of bone structures. It is the best modality for tumors of the tongue and is more sensitive for superficial tumors, detecting bone marrow invasion and it can be useful for evaluation of cartilage invasion. The latter advantage over CT scanning can be especially helpful. CT scanning is better than MRI for detection of bone cortex invasion, on the other hand. MRI is also considered the imaging technique of choice for perineural spread, skull base invasion, and intracranial extension of head and neck cancer. It is also great for base of tongue tumors and parotid gland lesions.

The main disadvantages include higher costs and longer acquisition time. The investigation is more complex with many possible sequences which can be performed and evaluation of the images is also more demanding. There are a multitude of potential artefacts (motion artefacts, flow artefacts, field distortion artefacts due to metal or at air bone interfaces or with blood products) which can mimic or obscure pathology. The face, neck and base of the skull have multiple soft tissue, air and bone interfaces with increased chance of susceptibility artefacts. Additionally movement and swallowing artefacts can degrade image quality. Examination of larger body areas is limited by longer duration of image acquisition. Gadolinium containing contrast agents should be given to evaluate tumours and abscesses. Contraindications to the use of gadolinium are absolute or relative and include previous or pre-existing nephrogenic systemic fibrosis (NSF), previous anaphylactic reaction to gadolinium containing contrast agents, patients with a glomerular filtration rate below 30 ml/min/1.73 square meter, unstable renal impairment, hepatorenal syndrome or chronic liver function disorders and pregnancy. Since macrocyclic compounds of gadolinium are known to be more stable than linear compounds of gadolinium, they should be preferably given if absolutely necessary.

There are also absolute and relative contraindications to performing MRI. A body weight over 200 kg precludes an MRI as the table cannot carry this weight. Other contraindications include ferromagnetic metal fragments near vital structures, metal implants in the area of interest, older pacemakers, nerve stimulators, pumps, cochlear implants and stapes prostheses, claustrophobia, very ill patients, patients who cannot lie down for long periods of time due to pain or increased risks of aspiration.

Increasingly the use of CT integrated PET scans is being acknowledged for various settings in the management of head and neck cancers. PET scan alone has unsatisfactory resolution, but nowadays mostly PET-CT is done. CT scan can be of low dose or of diagnostic quality, which makes a significant difference not only in resolution but also in the total radiation dose delivered. Many studies have proven that PET-CT scanning is comparable to conventional CT scans and MRI.

The advantages include evaluation of the whole body including the area of interest, lymph node involvement, detection and exclusion of distant metastases and the high sensitivity of detection of glucose uptake. One big disadvantage is that it is nonspecific as uptake is also increased in inflammation. It is also more expensive, time consuming, requires patient to be fasting for 6 hours, the scanning time is 20–30 minutes and the total investigation time is about 2–3 hours. There is some radiation exposure which varies depending on whether a low dose CT is done for attenuation correction or a diagnostic quality CT is performed. Interpretation can be difficult in areas of complex anatomy, physiological variants and unusual patterns of high FDG- uptake in the head and neck.

PET image evaluation is mainly performed by qualitative visual assessment. Visual assessment requires definition of a threshold for judgement of existence and degree of radiotracer concentration. A semi-quantitative parameter currently used for PET is the standardised uptake value, which is defined as the tissue concentration of tracer within a lesion divided by tissue density, as measured by PET, divided by the injected dose normalised to patient weight multiplied by a decay factor. Instead of body weight, the injected dose may also be corrected by the lean body mass, or body surface area (BSA). Different tumours also show different glucose uptake and there is no standard threshold value for diagnosis of tumours, however it can be useful for therapy monitoring.

A few studies have evaluated the role of PET-CT in finding out occult neck nodes but there is a lack of confidence about this modality replacing the need of an elective neck dissection. On the other hand, after definitive radiation, PET-CT negativity may be used as a surrogate marker for cure and neck dissection can be omitted.

The above mentioned modalities of imaging can not only be used for primary sites and lymph node mets but also for the discovery of occult systemic metastasis. The risk of occult metastasis depends on the primary site and clinical stage among other factors. The most common sites being lungs, liver and bones. Imaging studies have been consistently shown to be superior to tests like liver function tests, alkaline phosphatase and lactate dehydrogenase assay.

CHAPTER 6: PRINCIPLES OF RADIATION THERAPY AND COMBINED CHEMORADIATION

Radiation therapy offers cure at certain sites of head and neck cancers, with organ preservation. This could be achieved by radiation alone in early stages, and in combination with chemotherapy in locally advanced cases. Radiation therapy with or without chemo also has an important role to play in post-operative adjuvant settings, if high-risk features like advanced tumor stage (T3/T4), positive or close margins, two or more positive lymph nodes (N2/N3), extranodal extension and/or perineural or lymphovascular invasion are present. Postoperative concurrent chemoradiation should be used in cases with positive surgical margins or extranodal extension, while in the presence of other risk factors the addition of chemotherapy remains optional. Radiation offers palliation in advanced disease, like in the case of brain mets and painful bone metastasis et cetera.

Most commonly radiation in head and neck cancers is delivered by external beam; in rare cases brachytherapy in form of interstitial or intracavitary techniques may be used. External beam RT is delivered by linear accelerators in most of the centres worldwide. In these machines high energy electrons are generated that when collided with tungsten produce photons, which are then directed by the machine to the area of interest. In special circumstances, like skin tumors, the electrons themselves are used as they don't penetrate to deeper structures. The energy of photon beams thus generated is usually in the 4-6 megavolt range.

Planning of radiation delivery is the most crucial step. With modern CT scan machines cross sectional imaging is done and 2 to 3 mm slices are obtained for proper planning. A slice width above 5 mm is not acceptable. At certain sites like skull base, MRI may be more useful. Nowadays radiation machines come equipped with an inbuilt CT scanner.

The minimum required technique of head and neck radiation is 3D-CRT, anything below this level can't be used in modern practice as the results would be dismal. The standard-of-care worldwide is intensity modulated RT (IMRT). This technique is advantageous as the beam of energy here has varying intensities based upon the tumor characteristics and surrounding structures. Needless to say that to plan such a sophisticated radiation delivery needs expertise and there is a theoretical risk of missing the tumor volume. Another drawback of this technique is the time needed for delivery of radiation everyday is about 25 minutes, which can be problematic for patient convenience as well as prohibitive for treating a large number of patients on a single machine, which often is the case in practice. Newer techniques like VMAT circumvent this problem and using the arc this technology finishes the delivery in less than 5 minutes.

In many centres worldwide, image guided RT is increasingly used. The advantages are daily imaging, which leads to less error and lesser toxicity to surrounding tissues. The reason for improved accuracy using this technique are millimeter changes that inevitably happen as patients position ever so slightly varies under the machine daily.

There are many fractionation schedules available for delivery of desired radiation dose. One such approach, which uses more than one fraction per day (hyperfractionation) has shown benefit in overall survival compared with conventional fractionation in some trials; whereas "accelerated" one did not. The small benefit in overall survival and the logistic challenges in giving more than one fraction daily, coupled with cost considerations make hyperfractionation problematic to adopt as standard.

Recently, proton and carbon ion therapies are coming to the fore. These have unique physical properties, the most important of which is known as Bragg peak effect. Due to this property, the maximum effect occurs at the target site, while surrounding tissues are spared of toxicity. These modalities can be extremely helpful when the lesions are near critical structures like skull base and eye. The major issue remains the cost to the patient, not to mention the logistic problems regarding installing such expensive setup and the necessary training to facilitate maximal outcomes.

Brachytherapy has limited role in head and neck cancer management, as opposed to certain other sites like cervix and endometrial cancer where it has a major role to play. Most of the times it is used as boost and in a select few patients, criteria of selection of whom remain controversial; it could be used as a standalone modality.

Of course, the results of radiation therapy are not the same in every individual case. This is reflective of the varying degrees of sensitivity of different patients' cancerous cells to radiation induced cell killing. Some factors like high disease burden can be routinely predictive of the outcomes but most of the other mechanisms of "radioresistance" remain elusive in the absence of close scrutiny. Hypoxia is one of the biggest factors, as tissues which are hypoxic are more than twice as likely to show lesser response to radiation than oxygenated tissue. Differences in repopulation, p53 expression and ERCC-1 et cetera are other factors that contribute to differences in radiation sensitivity, hence outcomes.

Altering the schedules of radiation delivery, especially "hyperfractionation" and to some extent "accelerated" radiation schedules circumvent some problems like repopulation and can lead to improved survival outcomes. Correction of anemia is also beneficial for enhanced tumor cell kill. The most important strategy, though, remains addition of chemotherapy to radiation.

The mechanism of action of chemo given along with radiation are: Making DNA more susceptible to radiation damage and augmenting cell killing, interfering with DNA repair (cisplatin and gemcitabine), reduction of repopulation (hydroxyurea and fluorouracil), reducing the population of hypoxic tumor cells (mitomycin C), redistribution and accumulation of cells into the more radiosensitive G2 and M phases (taxanes) among others.

Hence, although radiation can be curative alone in certain early stage head and neck cancers, in locoregionally advanced cancers and many times in the adjuvant setting as well, combination with chemotherapy is necessary. The idea behind this approach is that if chemo is given prior to radiation, it could shrink the tumor so that radiation field is then narrowed which leads to reduced toxicities. Chemo prior to radiation also has the potential to work on distant metastasis. When chemo is given along with radiation, known as concurrent chemoradiation, it has the potential to sensitize the cancerous cells to radiation, resulting in enhanced tumor cell death. Also concurrent chemo, as it's cytotoxic, leads to reduction in the "repopulation" of malignant cells between radiation fractions. The third method, known as "sequential" chemoradiotherapy combines both chemo given before and during the radiation course.

Multiple trials have been done on the subject of combination chemoradiotherapy versus radiation or surgery alone. A seminal meta-analysis of which has shown that across all major head and neck cancer sites (nasopharyngeal cancers were not a part of this meta-analysis) combined chemoradiation compared with local therapies alone (surgery or radiation) results in 6.5 percent absolute decrease in mortality at five years.

Comparing different chemotherapy integration approaches, concurrent chemotherapy and induction chemotherapy followed by definitive therapy comparison is a difficult topic. The consensus is to use concurrent chemo with radiation. Local control rates are better with concurrent therapy whereas induction chemo is considered more effective for distant metastasis. The relative value of each approach, of course, depends on the primary site and patient related factors. The time interval between completion of induction chemo and starting of radiation should be after 3 weeks and within 5 weeks.

Sequential chemoradiation combines the best of both worlds, at least in theory. But the data suggests otherwise, as multiple trials done on the subject of comparison between sequential and concurrent methods have failed to show any significant survival benefit, although some trials showed reduction in distant mets with the former.

In the past, cisplatin and infusional 5-FU were used as induction chemo. Later, trials established the triplet of cisplatin, 5-FU and a taxane as the standard induction. Concurrent chemoradiotherapy protocols employ high-dose bolus cisplatin (100 mg/m_2 on days 1, 22, and 43) as the gold standard, but this is associated with limiting toxicities. Many centres worldwide use cisplatin 40 mg/m^2 weekly to address the toxicity while maintaining efficacy. Carboplatin is an alternative in poor performance status patients and patients who are not candidates for cisplatin. Cetuximab may be an option, for poor performance status patients albeit with reduced efficacy; and it may not be a good option for patients who are not candidates for chemotherapy as a whole because of their general condition.

At the end of radiation (with or without chemotherapy), assessment is made for residual tumor and if the desired response is not attained then surgical salvage is to be done. The time difference between completion of radiation and assessment of response should be 10 to 12 weeks but some experts recommend 6 to 8 weeks, if the residual tumor is grossly there.

Patients who present with neck nodes and are treated with radiation as primary modality pose a challenge. In the past there were criteria that mandated neck dissection in patients who fit these criteria, regardless of response. Nowadays with improved imaging techniques, observation is the first choice. Patients are clinically assessed routinely and if they show no sign of progression by week 4 to 6, observation is continued and by week 12 a PET-CT scan (preferably) is done. If PET-

CT shows no avid residual tumor, then observation is continued. In case the findings are equivocal then repeat PET-CT is done 4 to 6 weeks later, if it still remains equivocal or progression is there, then salvage surgery is done. If the PET-CT done by week 12 shows progression then salvage surgery is done.

Some patients show a mixed picture, in them PET component of the scan is normal but CT scan still shows a residual mass. In such cases the risk status is assessed. Low risk patients are those who have theoretical low risk of having residual cancer like those of HPV associated oropharyngeal carcinoma, having received optimum treatment. Patients who have had treatment interruptions and those with other than oropharyngeal primaries should be considered high risk. If the patient belongs to the high risk category then 2 to 3 monthly clinical and imaging examinations are done, if there is progression at anytime salvage surgery is undertaken. In low risk patients clinical surveillance alone is done, without imaging.

The extent of the surgery to be done depends upon the primary site and the clinical context. More is not better in this case and selective neck dissection should be done whenever possible; as more extensive neck dissections don't improve survival in such patients while adding unnecessary morbidity.

Reirradiation:

Upto half of the patients treated with radiation, as a curative modality, may develop recurrence; either local or distant. These recurrences ought to be managed by salvage surgery whenever feasible theoretically and if the patient's general condition is permissive of the potentially high-risk and morbid surgery; and if not then reirradiation is an alternative. Re-RT is also needed if pathology report after surgical salvage shows high-risk features.

As a general rule, recurrences that develop within the first six months of completion of primary radiation course are considered radioresistant and in these re-RT should not be done. In cases that develop after six months consideration is to be given to at risk structures like skin, nerves, blood vessels, and spinal cord; as they receive maximal tolerable radiation doses during the initial course and exposing these to any further radiation results in more than acceptable toxicity. So, the most precise methodology for delivery of radiation with margins no more than 2 cm should be undertaken.

Doses of more than 50 Gy have to be used to achieve meaningful outcomes and alternative fractionation schedules like hyperfractionation should play a role. Treatment of neck nodes poses a difficult challenge and most centres omit elective neck irradiation while treating the primary recurrence site.

Another controversial topic is debulking surgery prior to re-RT. Practice differs from centre to centre and in my opinion debulking surgery should be done whenever technically feasible, as long as it does not result in unacceptable morbidity.

Reirradiation should be combined with chemotherapy whenever medically feasible. Some experts suggest that the regimen of chemotherapy used during the primary radiation course should not be used, although this is more of a mere opinion than a scientifically proven fact. Combination of hydroxyurea and 5-FU has been studied very well with good results. Adding another drug like a taxane may be additive to the effect. In some cases, induction chemotherapy may be needed before re-RT. There is a severe dearth of studies in this aspect. Limited data suggest that induction with pemetrexed and gemcitabine followed by radiation with carboplatin and pemetrexed may be used. Now trials are ongoing that are studying the role of immunotherapy in combination with radiation. This may lead to a paradigm shift in the future as till now, the role of chemotherapy is that of a sensitizer to radiation; while the trials exploring the role of immunotherapy are suggesting the role of radiation as a sensitizer to immunotherapy molecules. Data are premature in this regard and we will have to wait.

Needless to say that acute and long-term complications are monumentally increased in reirradiated patients, as compared with those receiving radiation for the first time. But even then re-RT should be done, if it could be, as it provides a chance of cure.

CHAPTER 7: ORAL CAVITY

The boundaries of oral cavity are the skin-vermilion junction of the lips to the junction of the hard and soft palate above, and to the line of circumvallate papillae of the tongue below. The anterior tonsillar pillars and glossotonsillar folds serve as the lateral boundaries between the oral cavity and oropharynx.

The structures from which squamous cell carcinoma can arise in the oral cavity are the lip, floor of the mouth, oral tongue (anterior two-thirds of the tongue), lower alveolar ridge, upper alveolar ridge, retromolar trigone (retromolar gingiva), hard palate, and buccal mucosa. Other histologies can arise from other sites as well, but that's not the scope of this chapter.

The risk factor profile for this cancer is the same as we have discussed in a previous chapter. Smokeless tobacco has a huge impact on the development of oral cavity cancers, and ultraviolet light is a causative agent for lip cancers.

Staging of these cancers is done according to the AJCC system. The details of this staging system can be found on the AJCC website and text book.

Before starting treatment we must assess for tumor size, the extent or depth of invasion, and the regional lymph nodes. Oral cavity cancers tend to invade surrounding soft tissues early in their course, so it's important to incorporate imaging studies. CT scans are most frequently used, MRI is useful for tongue cancers and PET-CT scans are useful for local and distant metastasis evaluation.

For the sake of discussion, we will divide the oral cavity squamous cell carcinomas in early (stages one and two) and advanced (stages three and four). First we shall dwell on early stage oral cavity cancers.

As a general principle for stage one and two oral cavity cancers, surgery is preferred modality of treatment. Radiation may be used but only in cases where surgery is not considered feasible for any reason. There is no data backing this recommendation, and it reflects more of the cumulative clinical experience. Retromandibular trigone is a tricky site and radiation is often considered in the first line management.

For the early stage oral cavity cancers, traditional surgical approaches are most widely used. Robotic and other such techniques have become popular in other head and neck cancer sites but their utility in early stage oral cavity cancer is not of much magnitude. Obtaining negative margins is the primary objective in surgery of early stage head and neck cancers and if the final pathology report reveals positive or close (less than 5 mm) margins, then every attempt should be made for revision surgery. Complications can include infection, bleeding, aspiration, wound breakdown, flap loss, and fistula. The functional deficits may be there and will be discussed in the relevant section.

In tumors without deep invasion and lymphovascular invasion intraoral cone or interstitial brachytherapy may be used as a stand-alone modality. But these cases should be selected meticulously as these methods don't cover regional neck nodes.

Subsites in oral cavity squamous cell carcinomas:

Lips:

Cancers affecting the lips are most commonly the squamous and basal cell types. The etiology which is unique to these cancers among oral cavity cancers is ultraviolet light exposure. The treatment and prognosis is different depending upon whether the cancer has originated from the upper or lower lip.

Lower lip cancers are less prone to metastasize to lymph nodes and thus cure rates are higher. On the other hand, cancers involving the upper lip can spread to lymph nodes early and due to their vicinity to other vital structures may pose unique problems. For upper lip cancers, consideration is always given to treat the neck at the same time too.

Surgery is the preferred modality of treatment but in lip cancers there are unique challenges. Any surgical defect will be of cosmetic nature and in order to obtain a negative margin, sometimes reconstruction becomes necessary; not only for cosmetically accepted outcome but also to preserve functionality.

In general, the prognosis for early stage squamous cell carcinoma of the lip is very good, with 10-year recurrence-free survival rates of 94 and 78 percent for stage I and II disease, respectively.

Floor of mouth:

For these cancers due to high incidence of radiation induced toxicities, especially the ones affecting bones, surgery remains the preferred modality of treatment. Sometimes it becomes tricky and large defects may warrant reconstruction with flaps. One frequent iatrogenic complication is lingual nerve injury, which may be difficult to visualize. In a few studies done on this matter, results of radiation are comparable to that of surgery.

Five-year overall survival rates for stage I and II cancers of 95 and 85 percent have been reported.

Oral tongue:

Surgery is the appropriate first strategy, except for a small minority of patients who can be treated with brachytherapy. These cancers are especially prone to spread to lymph nodes of the neck and elective neck dissection is now recommended for most patients with tumors ≥3 mm thickness. Because of the frequent occurrence of "skip" metastasis, it is desirable to pursue a selective neck dissection of levels I to IV.

The prognosis of oral tongue cancers is variable, with large differences in studies. Five-year survival of 70 and 50 percent are cited for stage one and two patients respectively.

Retromolar trigone and lower alveolar ridge:

These cancers tend to be locally recurrent, primarily due to occult bone invasion, which may be left behind, giving spuriously negative margins; also there is a high probability of spread to regional nodes. Surgeries of retromandibular trigone can be very difficult, as obtaining a wide margin may warrant technically challenging defects.

Upper alveolar ridge and hard palate:

These cancers tend to stay localised and for this reason may have excellent prognosis. Surgery is preferred, although radiation yields similar results but at a cost of possibility of late toxicity.

Buccal mucosa:

Tumors of buccal mucosa are treated with surgery and as a general principle, reconstruction must be done, as not doing so will result in trismus. Surgeon has to balance the extent of surgery to maximize long term survival and disfigurement which is a function of the extent of the surgery. In most of the cases, post operative radiation with or without chemotherapy should be used.

Neck dissection: when and how?

In early stage oral cavity cancers, the management of neck is a controversial topic; it depends on the site as well. For example, in cancer of the tongue the rate of occult lymph node metastasis is higher, but that's not the case in hard palate cancers.

Tumor thickness is the deciding parameter upon which the management of neck rests. Previously a thickness of 4 mm was used as cutoff but now it has been revised to 3 mm, based on a large trial.

For patients with oral cavity cancer, it is recommended to perform an ipsilateral selective neck dissection, levels I to III/IV, for stage I cancers with greater than 3 mm of invasion and for most stage II disease. Levels IIB and IV are dissected at the discretion of the surgeon, beyond this level dissection is usually not necessary. Patients with primary tumors close to or involving the midline should be managed with bilateral neck dissection or sentinel lymph node biopsy.

In patients who are not treated by surgery, but instead by radiation therapy as a primary modality, the irradiation of neck follows the same principles as those of neck dissection.

Adjuvant radiation with or without chemo is indicated in patients with positive or close final resection margins, bone invasion, and for most patients with pathologically positive lymph nodes. Postoperative radiation therapy should be considered for depth of invasion and for tumor thickness >4 mm, even in the setting of a negative unilateral neck dissection, it should also be considered if there is lymphovascular or perineural invasion.

Now that we have discussed the early stage cancers of oral cavity, the discussion of advanced stage cancers is being undertaken. By definition, "advanced" are stage III and IV diseases having tumors greater than 4 cm in greatest dimension, invasion of adjacent structures, and/or evidence of lymph node involvement.

In these patients, imaging has a more important place as there are many times more chances of harboring distant metastasis, especially in the lungs. So, while CT or PET-CT scans can be performed in early stages; in advanced stages these are integral to management decision making.

Unlike the early stage cancers, these cancers involve all three modalities of cancer therapy, most of the times. Surgery should always be the first option, following which radiation or chemoradiation is employed to maximize chances of cure. RT and/or chemoradiotherapy are alternatives for patients who refuse surgery, have a technically unresectable tumor (eg, due to carotid artery encasement, vertebral or brain invasion, i.e., cT4b), would have an unacceptable functional outcome with surgery, or are medically inoperable.

Postoperative radiation therapy with or without concurrent chemotherapy is the standard of care for locoregionally advanced oral cavity cancers, as surgery alone leads to high recurrence rates. There may be exceptions like completely resected primary with a single lymph node, which has also been excised. If the patient is fit enough to tolerate, then chemotherapy should be used along with postoperative radiation therapy. To be more specific, the risk factors that confer a high risk of recurrence include extranodal extension, positive resection margins, N2 or N3 nodal disease, nodal disease in levels IV or V, perineural invasion, or vascular invasion. For positive margins and extranodal extension chemoradiotherapy is indicated while the other factors suggest that chemo should be added. If none of these risk factors is present then postoperative radiation alone is indicated.

In some patients, the operability is borderline. In these patients the idea of giving chemotherapy before surgery, thus reducing the growth sufficiently to make it amenable to surgery and thus improving outcomes, seems very attractive. This strategy is known as induction chemotherapy and while on paper there is nothing wrong with this idea, the two large trials done in this regard have failed to show improvement in survival. Having said that, these trials showed reduction in the extent and the morbidity caused by surgery and the need of postoperative radiation was also reduced. This strategy should only be used in a select few cases after a thorough multidisciplinary discussion.

Some patients can't undergo surgery either due to personal preference, medical comorbidities that prohibit undertaking surgery or due to unresectable tumor like those with carotid artery encasement, vertebral or brain invasion. In such patients, combined chemoradiotherapy is the first option, unless the patient is not fit enough to tolerate chemotherapy concurrently, in which case radiation alone may be employed. Another approach is to use induction chemotherapy followed by radiation with or without chemo, this approach should be taken only after multidisciplinary discussion as radiation fields may need to be altered according to disease at presentation and response upon evaluation may be challanging.

Locally advanced cancers of the oral cavity either have nodal involvement at presentation, in which case they have to be addressed as per the situation; or there may not be discernible nodes, but the chances of occult mets being present is sufficiently high in most of the cases, warranting neck node management on an elective basis.

A selective dissection including levels I to III, a supraomohyoid neck dissection, is typically sufficient for clinically N0 oral cavity cancer, as level IV and V nodes are rarely involved without clinical disease at other levels. This dissection includes the submandibular gland but preserves the spinal accessory nerve, the internal jugular vein, and the sternocleidomastoid muscle. In oral tongue cancers, however, due to the possibility of "skip metastasis", level IV is also dissected.

Patients who have clinical involvement of neck nodes to present with, modified radical neck dissection is usually performed; although selective neck dissection in expert hands has shown equal oncological outcomes.

The management of contralateral neck depends on the tumor site and proximity to midline. Expert opinion varies, but the consensus seems to be around the fact that if the tumor is near midline at certain sites, bilateral neck dissection should be done followed by radiation. Some centres give radiation alone, and no surgery, to the other side of neck if no nodes can be clinically identified.

CHAPTER 8: OROPHARYNX

The subsites from which oropharyngeal cancers can arise are: soft palate, tonsils, base of tongue, pharyngeal wall, and vallecula. This disease has a peculiar epidemiology. Conventionally, smoking and alcohol were considered the main etiological factors; but in countries where smoking rates gradually declined, the incidence of oropharyngeal cancers rose. Later, the correlation was made between this and human papilloma virus infection.

The biology of the squamous cell carcinoma arising due to tobacco and alcohol is different from those of HPV induced. HPV associated oropharyngeal carcinoma have a better prognosis and less intensive protocols may deliver equal oncological outcomes. This formed the basis of the latest AJCC staging system update for these cancer, which now divides them into HPV related (p16 positive) oropharyngeal carcinoma and p16 negative tumors of the oropharynx. Under this new classification scheme, HPV related oropharyngeal primary with neck node involvement can be classified as early stage compared with the fact that in patients with non-HPV related cancers the involvement of neck nodes confers a stage four designation.

First we will discuss the early stage oropharyngeal cancers. Surgery and radiation, as standalone modalities give equal oncological outcomes. The choice of surgery is most of the times between transoral robotic surgery and transoral laser microsurgery. Radiation without chemotherapy is recommended in early stage cancers.

As a general rule, the cancers of oropharynx have the propensity to spread to cervical lymph nodes; and that too bilaterally. This is partly due to the fact that this area has especially rich lymphatic network and also due to anatomical positioning which frequently results in breach of midline. Hence, management of neck is imperative even in the early stages. Generally, bilateral neck nodes should be addressed either by radiation or by neck dissection. There are subtle differences according to the anatomic subsites, which we will now discuss.

Early stage soft palate cancers are most of the

time treated with RT, as surgery is associated with more functional deficits compared with radiation. When treating with RT, bilateral neck node irradiation should be done.

Tonsillar cancers are mostly taken up for surgery. Previously, open surgeries were done but with the advent of robotic and laser techniques, the surgeries have become way less morbid, with excellent functional outcomes. Even in advanced stages these cancers have a good prognosis, as they are most commonly associated with HPV. Radiation can be used with equal oncological outcomes.

Base of tongue needs special consideration, as it has got the highest probability of occult lymph node mets among subsites of oropharynx. Upto half of the patients with apparent early stage base of tongue cancers may harbor occult lymph node mets. In practice, radiation therapy is used as a primary modality; although evolution of surgical techniques have now made surgeries of this region feasible, which used to be very morbid in the past. Overall, it's tricky site to operate on and final pathology report after surgery many times still necessitates radiation which results in further morbidity. Bilateral neck should always be addressed with the modality being used for the treatment of the primary site.

After the primary treatment is over, further adjuvant therapy may be needed. If the patient was treated with radiation primarily and the disease is not showing complete response then surgery should be done for salvage. If patient was treated with surgery initially and the final pathology shows positive margins or extranodal extension, adjuvant chemoradiation is indicated. Other features may tilt the clinical decision making towards adjuvant therapy and these should be individualised.

Now coming to the locoregionally advanced oropharyngeal cancers, one issue ought to be dealt with first. In the latest edition of AJCC staging for head and neck cancer, many significant changes have been made with regard to oropharyngeal cancers. It will be important to note here that the treatment decision making is still done on the basis of the previous edition of AJCC. Hence, some patients who are locoregionally advanced but HPV (p16) positive, will be categorised as stage one or two but these will still be treated as if they are locoregionally advanced, and not like the early stage cancers, however their designation might be.

The principles of oncology, namely "primum non nocere" and "hasten to help" apply to the treatment of these cancers as well. The first priority is to do no harm, and for this purpose organ preserving methods are first opted. In locally advanced oropharyngeal cancers, radiation combined with chemotherapy is most often used. Although in some patients who have small primaries surgery may be done followed by radiation, primarily to reduce dose of radiation.

The rationale of combining chemotherapy with radiation comes from a meta-analysis of trials which concluded that the chemotherapy combination with radiation corresponded to an absolute improvement of 5 percent in overall survival at five years and 8 percent when the chemotherapy was given concurrently. In larynx cancer, there is a debate about the proper role of induction chemotherapy but in the case of oropharyngeal cancers, there appears to be no role of this approach, as far as survival outcomes are concerned. In a select few induction chemo followed by radiation therapy may be used but there is no solid foundation for such a practice.

The most commonly used regimen in combined modality therapy is cisplatin 100 mg/m^2 every 3 weekly with radiation. Many other protocols have been studied and can be used depending on the clinical situation. The notion that HPV positive cancer treatment protocols may forego of cisplatin, using cetuximab in lieu of it; was disproved in a recent clinical trial. So cisplatin remains the gold standard.

Surgery has a somewhat controversial role in the management of locoregionally advanced oropharyngeal cancers. The surgeries required after morbid and many a times warrant further adjuvant chemoradiation nevertheless; so surgery should be chosen as primary treatment modality only after thorough multidisciplinary discussion.

When radiation is used as primary treatment, bilateral neck node irradiation is warranted, and if there is lack of adequate response after radiation then surgery ought to be done. In a few select patients, in whom surgery is done first, most of the times bilateral neck dissection is required in the locoregionally advanced oropharyngeal cancers. In some cases of N0 or N1 disease, selective neck dissection may provide equally good oncological outcomes with less morbidity compared with modified radical neck dissection.

CHAPTER 9: HYPOPHARYNX

The superior boundary of the hypopharynx is formed by the oropharynx at the level of the hyoid bone and the inferior boundary is marked by the esophageal inlet at the lower end of the cricoid cartilage. It is divided in three subsites of which pyriform sinus is the subsite out of which most of the cancers of hypopharynx arise. Posterior pharyngeal wall and post cricoid space are the other two subsites.

These cancers are seldom detected early due to lack of symptoms at early stages. Presenting symptoms can include dysphagia, odynophagia, otalgia, hoarseness, dyspnea or stridor with or without a neck mass. They tend to spread to the draining lymph nodes early on in the course and distant metastasis are also not uncommon. Approximately two thirds have neck node involvement and one fifth have distant metastasis at presentation.

Smoking and chewing tobacco and alcohol consumption are the main risk factors. Iron deficiency in its extreme scenario leads to Plummer-Vinson syndrome, which is a risk factor unique to these cancers.

As these tumors do not produce symptoms in the early stages, they are not usually detected when they are stage one or two. But if they are detected, either due to a minority of these cancers produce symptoms or due to some routine examination directed at some other complaint, then evaluation should be done. Fiberoptic examination and imaging studies (vide supra) are utilized to reach at a proper staging evaluation.

Treatment:

As hypopharynx is located at a critical juncture, radical surgical approach should not be taken in early stage cancers. Radiation therapy is the most commonly used modality, results of which are comparable to surgery with less morbidity. Organ preserving surgeries can be used and follow the same principles as in larynx. One important distinction is, as we have already discussed, that the possibility of occult neck node mets is higher in hypopharynx; so neck management is imperative. If radiation is used then neck should be covered and the same goes for surgery as well.

If surgery is used to treat the primary tumor, bilateral selective neck dissection of levels II, III, and IV should be performed for patients who present with clinically negative necks. For patients who undergo definitive RT to the primary tumor the entire bilateral neck, including the retropharyngeal and supraclavicular nodes, generally should be part of the treatment volume, even in patients with early tumors and clinically negative neck nodes.

As far as stage three and four (locally advanced) hypopharynx cancers are concerned; many of the trials done on the subject have taken patients of both larynx and hypopharynx cancers combined and the principles and the methods of management of both these cancer sites are identical. So the reader is requested to refer the section of management of advanced laryngeal cancers, as the same holds true for hypopharynx cancers as well.

CHAPTER 10: LARYNX

Worldwide, there are an estimated 250,000 cases of laryngeal cancer and 100,000 deaths annually. This disease primarily affects men, partly due to differences in smoking habits.

Anatomy of the larynx:

It is divided into three regions: the supraglottis, glottis, and subglottis:

Supraglottis includes suprahyoid epiglottis, infrahyoid epiglottis, aryepiglottic folds, arytenoids, and false cords; glottis has true vocal cords, including anterior and posterior commissures, subglottis is constituted of the area, extending from lower boundary of the glottis to the lower margin of the cricoid cartilage. Cancers of glottis constitute two thirds of all larynx cancers.

First we will discuss the management of "early" laryngeal cancers, i.e., stage one and two. The goal of the treatment in early laryngeal cancers is preservation of function (also known as organ preservation approach) which are: airway patency, occlusion of the airway during swallowing, and phonation. These should be viewed in conjunction with the overarching principles of cancer management, most important of which is survival endpoint benefit.

Surgery and radiation are equally effective modalities as far as oncological outcomes are concerned. But surgery (larynx preservation surgery) is less desirable as functional outcomes are better preserved with radiation therapy. In these patients chemotherapy should be combined with radiation therapy only in very selected scenarios, as otherwise there is no benefit and only added toxicity is there. In most cases, total laryngectomy is unnecessary as radical radiotherapy techniques are used in lieu of surgery.

Larynx-preserving surgical techniques are partial open laryngectomy, transoral laser microsurgery (using carbon dioxide laser, although newer options are coming to the fore), and transoral robotic surgery. These approaches are safe in experienced hands but if confidence is not there then it's better to go for radiation as in case of inadequately performed surgery, post operative radiation is nevertheless needed and then the functional outcome will not be as good as in the case of radiation having been used as a standalone therapy.

There are differences in treatment approaches depending upon the subsite involved within the larynx. In both glottic and supraglottic cancers, the primary tumor is best treated with preferably radiation therapy alone, or with the help of larynx-preserving surgery; but neck nodes are not usually treated in glottis cancers whereas in supraglottic cancers are prone to metastasize to neck, due to their rich lymphatic network, so in these cases neck nodes must be treated even in early stage cancers. Subglottic cancers are very rare but they are the most aggressive of the subset and often total laryngectomy is contemplated due to anticipated poor outcomes of the other treatment approaches, neck must also be addressed in these tumors all the time.

Locally advanced laryngeal cancers:

Patients of larynx cancers of stage III and IV are advanced cancers, in this section we will discuss the management of these cancers, except those with distant metastasis. Radiation combined with chemotherapy is the most commonly used approach as it has the potential to spare function with equal oncological outcomes compared with radical surgical approach of total laryngectomy. Although in selected cases function preserving surgical approaches, like in the case of early cancers may also be used but it is important to note here that none of these approaches have been compared with each other.

Combined modality therapy employs chemotherapy given at the same time as RT (*concurrent* chemoradiotherapy), *induction* chemotherapy followed by RT without chemotherapy, or *sequential* therapy with induction chemotherapy followed by concurrent chemoradiotherapy. In patients who are unfit to receive chemotherapy, radiation alone can be used albeit with compromise in survival outcomes.

Combined chemoradiotherapy approaches are not suitable for all patients due to a variety of reasons. Elderly patients with poor performance status or compromised end organ function are not good candidates for combination of chemoradiation, in these patients radiation alone or laryngectomy followed by radiation may be more tolerable. Patients, in whom bilateral vocal cords have become irreversibly damaged, derive no literal benefit of the "organ preserving approaches"; in them surgery should be the way to go, as the relief of symptoms would be permanent and the

HEAD AND NECK CANCER

toxicity will be considerably less. Cartilage invasion is a controversial topic, as it seriously hampers the potential recovery post chemoradiotherapy and many experts believe that surgery should be undertaken as the primary treatment; while another school of thought considers chemoradiation first and surgical salvage later, if needed.

The basis of these recommendations came from carefully performed randomized controlled trials, the most important ones of which being Department of Veterans Affairs (VA) Laryngeal Cancer Study Group larynx trial and European cooperative group trial (EORTC 24891). In the VA study patients were randomised between three cycles of induction chemotherapy with cisplatin plus fluorouracil, followed by definitive RT or primary surgery followed by postoperative RT. At a median follow-up of 33 months, the two-year survival rate was equal in both treatment groups, while larynx was preserved in around two thirds of patients on the chemo followed by RT arm. The european trial also showed equal oncological outcomes with both of the above mentioned treatment approaches while preserving laryngeal function with the organ preservation approach after a follow-up of ten years.

One interesting finding of RTOG trial was that in the arm of combination concurrent chemoradiation, there were more deaths, nature of which remained inexplicable. Further trials were done on the subject of concurrent chemoradiation versus induction chemotherapy followed by radiation alone, the results of which have been not very clear. Then finally a meta-analysis was done, which conclusively showed overall survival outcomes in favor of concurrent chemoradiation, thus establishing this approach as a standard-of-care. Guidelines recommend concurrent chemoradiotherapy for good performance status patients with resectable, locally advanced (stage III and carefully selected stage IV) laryngeal cancer, with a platinum-based chemotherapy regimens, such as cisplatin in a dose of 100 mg/m^2 every three weeks.

The subject of induction chemo versus concurrent chemo is a very controversial one. In RTOG trial there were more unexplained deaths in concurrent chemo arm, the overall survival were not different though. In a subsequent meta-analysis, there were no differences in survival outcomes between these two approaches, but when cisplatin and infusional 5-FU was used as induction chemo, survival was improved. A further trial which compared cisplatin and infusional 5-FU with the same combination coupled with a taxane, the survival outcomes were further improved. An important consideration is the patterns of recurrence. With concurrent chemo there *weren't* more distant failures whereas with induction chemo local recurrences were higher. Overall, it's not easy to choose one over another and patients should be informed of the choices available. Clinical situation, physician preference and individual centre based guidelines should play a greater role than simply choosing one approach blindly.

Another strategy would be to use induction chemotherapy followed by concurrent chemoradiotherapy (sequential). In theory this approach seems attractive, as it combines the best of two worlds: reduction in distant failures and decreased local recurrences. But with the exception of TAX 324 trial and an Italian trial, no phase three trial done till date has been able to show a survival benefit of this method. In select patients, it can be used, after multidisciplinary discussion.

In patients who have poor performance status, multiple comorbidities and limited natural life expectancy; surgery may be used as primary treatment modality in advanced cancers of the larynx. Surgery can be radical, namely total laryngectomy, or larynx-preservation surgery using trans-oral laser, open cervical or other such approaches may be an option. Surgery is needed in patients whose disease is not eradicated with chemoradiotherapy.

Neck management poses a challenge in cases of

larynx cancer. Cancers affecting glottis tend to **not** spread to neck nodes due to the scare lymphatic supply of this region; on the other hand, cases of supraglottis and especially subglottis are prone to metastasize to neck.

Management of neck is obviously dependent upon the primary modality chosen. When chemoradiation is used, usually observation is done, even in patients who presented with neck nodes. Serial monitoring is done with PET-CT scans and in case of persistent adenopathy or progression, neck dissection is performed.

If the patient is treated with surgery as the initial approach then bilateral prophylactic selective neck dissection, including levels II to IV, is recommended for patients with T3 and T4 tumors with clinically negative cervical nodes (N0) or early nodal disease (N1). RT is an alternative treatment for patients with N0 or N1 lymph nodes, particularly if the primary site requires adjuvant RT.

In patients who are managed by surgery and have clinically positive lymph nodes, neck dissection is done; particularly is cases of N2 or N3 disease modified radical neck dissection is done. In carefully chosen patients, selective neck dissection can be done to preserve cosmesis and prevent the development of complications like lymphedema.

Patients who are treated with surgery and in whom total laryngectomy is undertaken, face unique challenges. This procedure is often considered in frail elderly patients, anticipated to not tolerate chemoradiation well. Advantages are immediate relief of symptoms, reduction or elimination of aspiration and shorter treatment course.

The major challenge faced is the loss of voice function. For this, there are many rehabilitative techniques available. One such method employs electrical stimulation via a handheld device, known as artificial larynx or electrolarynx. The speech can be well understood which is thus produced, but the mechanical quality of voice is unacceptable to many individuals.

Another method is to create a fistula in the wall between esophagus and trachea. In expert hands this technique is incredibly effective. Care has to be taken to avoid so many complications that can easily arise.

The third method is called the esophageal speech, in it the patient "swallows" the air into the esophagus and liberates it to produce sound. This is a difficult trick to learn and the quality and loudness of the sound is inferior compared to the aforementioned methods.

CHAPTER 11:
NASOPHARYNX

Carcinoma of nasopharynx are a distinct subset among head and neck cancer sites. Many aspects of this malignancy are unique; ranging from etiology, histology, staging groups, treatment protocols and prognosis. Histologically it is divided into three major types which are: keratinizing squamous cell carcinoma (WHO type I), nonkeratinizing carcinoma, including differentiated (WHO type II) and undifferentiated carcinoma (WHO type III). Other subtypes are also there but they are rare.

The staging is done in accordance with the eighth edition of AJCC and there are many subtle differences in the eighth edition compared with the seventh edition, for which the reader is requested to refer to the appropriate text. The stage groups that have conventionally helped in clinical decision making are early, intermediate and advanced. As a general rule RT alone is sufficient for early stages, RT in combination with concurrent chemo is used for intermediate stages and for advanced stage concurrent chemoradiotherapy coupled with adjuvant chemotherapy or in some cases, induction chemotherapy is used. The current standard of care for concurrent chemotherapy is cisplatin either 100 mg/m2 on days 1, 22, and 43 or a weekly dose of 30 to 40 mg/m2.

Nasopharynx is anatomically a prohibitive site for surgery as the first line treatment. Although some centres may perform radical procedures like nasopharyngectomy in select cases but that's not the norm. In most cases radiation therapy in form of external beam at total doses of 70 to 72 Gray to the primary tumor and 50 Gy to the uninvolved neck in single daily fractions of 2 Gy, five days per week over six to seven weeks is often used for early stages. In intermediate or advanced stage, the primary tumor dose remains the same but the dose to the neck is increased to 66 to 70 Gy. One important principle ought to be emphasized here that because nasopharyngeal cancers have a high propensity to spread to neck nodes, bilateral neck irradiation has to be done, even in cases with clinically negative necks. Although in early stage cancers with clinically negative necks, irradiation of supraclavicular nodes could be omitted.

Apart from this conventional dosing schedule other strategies like hyperfractionation and accelerated delivery are also studied and may be used in an appropriate clinical context. Among histological subtypes of nasopharyngeal cancer, undifferentiated type is the most radiosensitive and keratinizing type is the least; which also reflects on their respective prognosis. That being said, the role of EBV positivity on prognosis prediction is less clear and some trials have been done in which stratification of patients according to EBV status and tailoring of therapy accordingly, especially adjuvant chemotherapy after completion of radiation was studied with nonsignificant results.

In advanced but not distant metastatic patients, adjuvant chemotherapy has a role. Trials done on this subject have shown improved outcomes when adjuvant chemotherapy was used; but in those pivotal trials the two arms were concurrent chemoradiotherapy followed by adjuvant chemotherapy versus radiation therapy alone. So in the modern era where concurrent chemoradiation is routinely used, the effect of chemotherapy in the adjuvant setting is less clear. Nevertheless, adjuvant chemotherapy is given in these clinical settings.

Recurrences:

Locally recurrent cases may have prolonged survival in some instances. Many models have been developed for the prediction of course of the disease in these patients. Reirradiation and salvage surgery are options and the choice between these two is dictated by clinical factors, like response and duration of response to prior RT; anatomical consideration; patient factors et cetera. Nasopharyngectomy is an option, but in recurrent cases the anatomical boundaries are breached as a routine and previous radiation may make obtaining surgical planes difficult. Newer surgical techniques like robotic surgery and newer radiation techniques like proton and carbon ion therapy may be beneficial.

If surgery is undertaken then further adjuvant radiation or combined chemoradiation may be needed based on the final pathology report and other risk factors.

Distant metastasis:

In patients who are medically fit enough, the combination of cisplatin and gemcitabine is considered the best based on an RCT. Otherwise nasopharyngeal cancer is considered a very chemosensitive malignancy and a wide range of chemotherapy molecules are effective.

In some patients who have the so called "oligometastatic" disease (the number and location of such limited metastasis is not defined); distant sites could be tackled by radiation or surgery or chemotherapy and the primary site undergoes a radical approach, thus giving the patient a chance of cure.

In case the patient is not fit to receive cisplatin then substitution with carboplatin or alteration of dose schedule may be an option; as can be the usage of other chemo molecules depending on the clinical factors.

A wide number of novel therapies are being studied, some of which have shown promising results, although most of the trials have been phase two and further data are needed before making recommendations. Small molecule tyrosine kinase inhibitors, anti-EGFR antibodies, cytotoxic T lymphocytes, pembrolizumab, nivolumab et cetera are being actively investigated.

CHAPTER 12: SALIVARY GLAND TUMORS

These are rare malignancies. For practical purposes, tumors may arise from major (parotid, submandibular and sublingual) and minor salivary glands. Parotid gland is most commonly involved, although the majority of tumors arising from parotid are benign. In contrast, tumors arising from other glands are mostly malignant.

The most common benign salivary gland tumor is pleomorphic adenoma and the most common malignant ones are mucoepidermoid carcinoma and adenoid cystic carcinoma. A wide variety of other histologies can also arise from salivary glands. In general these tumors are considered to be prone to local recurrence and distant metastasis.

The etiology of these tumors is not well defined. "Conventional" risk factors for head and neck cancers like tobacco and alcohol don't seem to play a major role in the development of salivary gland tumors. Occupational exposures, radiation and viruses have been implicated albeit with not strong causal relations.

A painless mass is the most common presentation. With increasing extent of the mass, surrounding structures may be compressed leading to correlating symptoms, for example, entrapment of nerves and the ensuing neuropathy.

Clinical examination, CT scan and MRI scan (both may sometimes be necessary) and ultrasound of the neck help stage the disease and the tissue diagnosis is imperative before treatment decision making as many of these masses are actually benign or may be histologies that have very different treatment options from each other. For this purpose biopsy or fine needle aspiration can be used as both methods have a high yield and accuracy.

If the tumor is technically resectable and the patient is medically fit to undergo the procedure, then surgery is the most appropriate treatment. In cases of benign lesions, surgery alone is sufficient; whereas in malignant lesion adjuvant therapy may be needed based on the risk factors. It is important to note here that most of these recommendations are based on clinical experiences, as randomised trial data is not there to guide decision making.

Parotid gland tumors:

It can't be emphasized enough that "simple enucleation" is not an adequate procedure for parotid gland tumors, or for any other salivary gland tumor, whether the tumor is benign or malignant. Parotidectomy can be of many types, depending upon the nature of mass and its extent, but most importantly, its relation with the facial nerve. When the facial nerve is not fully dissected, parotidectomy is called "conservative or partial". When dissection is done along all the branches of the facial nerve, superficial lobe is resected but deep lobe is not resected, it's known as "superficial". And when both the lobes are dissected, but preserving the facial nerve then it's known as "total". As is apparent from this discussion, preservation of the facial nerve is of prime importance, regardless of the extent of surgery; even if it leads to positive margins with respect to facial nerve.

As a general rule, most of the benign tumors of parotid require superficial parotidectomy and most of the malignant tumors require total parotidectomy; but these could be modified depending on the clinical situation. Malignant tumors that penetrate the deep structures may require extensive procedures like mandibulectomy et cetera. Many such procedures may yield positive margins.

Submandibular gland tumors:

In contrast with parotid gland tumors, majority of the submandibular gland tumors are malignant. Surgery is the mainstay of the treatment. Special consideration, regarding their preservation, must be given to vital structures that lie in the vicinity of these tumors including facial artery and vein, the marginal mandibular branch of the facial nerve, the hypoglossal and lingual nerves, and Wharton duct.

The principles of management of sublingual glands remain aligned with the rest of salivary gland tumors, surgery being the cornerstone of treatment. Neck dissection may need to be done on a higher index of suspicion for these tumors.

Minor salivary gland tumors:

There are hundreds to thousands of minor salivary glands distributed throughout head and neck mucosa, their highest concentration is found on the hard palate. Depending on the site of involvement, radiation therapy may be used as the first and standalone therapy but surgery followed (or not) by radiation is the most appropriate treatment whenever possible.

Neck management:

When there is clinical involvement of neck nodes and surgery is being done at the primary site and intention is *not* to give adjuvant radiation to the primary salivary gland tumor site; then selective neck dissection should be performed. In cases where radiation in electively being planned for the primary site in the postoperative setting, then expert opinion is divided on performing an elective neck dissection as well for the clinically positive neck.

The management of clinically negative neck is controversial and for some subsites like sublingual gland malignancies, neck dissection may be electively undertaken, especially if flaps are used for reconstruction.

The cases which are primarily managed by radiation, due to whatever reasons, neck nodes may be electively covered by radiation. Although in the face of lack of trial data, general recommendations are hard to make.

Adjuvant therapy:

For benign salivary gland tumors, adjuvant therapy has no definite role. Most of the times it's unnecessary, but some patients of pleomorphic adenoma who have positive margins and other high risk features may be taken for post operative radiation. This, of course, is very controversial.

Tumors that have large size (T3/T4), positive margins, positive overlying skin and related nerve(s), among other risk factors, are candidates for post operative radiation therapy. Chemotherapy is most of the times not needed, but as has been pointed out earlier; the lack of randomized trial data prohibits making general rules. So, in some cases chemotherapy may be added. Although chemotherapy alone has no role in the adjuvant setting.

Locally recurrent disease:

Surgery offers the best chance of cure in locoregionally recurrent cases. Even if the disease has become metastatic, surgery offers the best palliation at the local recurrence site. After surgery, adjuvant radiation is most of the times needed. In cases where surgery is not possible, radiation with or without chemotherapy may be used. If neither is possible then chemotherapy is a last resort, the principles of which are outlined under the following topic.

Metastatic disease:

The treatment of metastatic disease is dependent

on the clinical context. While some metastatic patients may just be observed, if they are not overtly symptomatic. On the other hand, a select few patients with oligometastatic disease could be treated with intent to achieve long term cure. Most of the times, the treatment remains palliative and the effect of chemotherapy on the prolongation of survival is not known; and as per the clinical observations, isn't very apparent.

A combination of cisplatin, doxorubicin and cyclophosphamide is most widely used, and should be the combination of choice if the patient is fit enough to tolerate. If that is not the case, then a wide variety of cytotoxic chemotherapy molecules are there that show clinical activity. Paclitaxel is very effective against adenocarcinomas and mucoepidermoid carcinomas but not adenoid cystic carcinomas.

There are many other newer options like larotrectinib for NTRK expressing tumors, trastuzumab (in combination with chemotherapy) for mucoepidermoid carcinomas and salivary duct cancers overexpressing human epidermal growth factor 2 (HER2) and androgen inhibitors for androgen receptor expressing salivary duct carcinomas. Drugs like imatinib for c-kit mutation; gefitinib and cetuximab for EGFR have failed to show benefit.

CHAPTER 13: PARANASAL SINUSES, NASAL CAVITY AND NASAL VESTIBULE

Paranasal sinuses: A number of different malignancies can arise from maxillary, ethmoid, sphenoid and frontal sinuses. Adenocarcinoma and squamous cell carcinoma are the most common of these histologies. Maxillary sinus is the most commonly affected. Apart from tobacco, factors like wood dust, certain heavy metals and some other occupational agents can give rise to these cancers.

Symptomatology of these tumors is dependent upon the site of involvement and the degree of involvement of the surrounding structures. Facial asymmetry, visible tumor are local effects. When it begins to encroach orbit and nerves, other symptoms start to appear.

The first step in diagnosis is biopsy of the lesion, which could often only be done by endoscopy; although transnasal approaches may be employed. If tumor is grossly visualized in the oral cavity then biopsy may be done from there as well.

For delineation of the local extent of the tumor, CT scan and/or MRI scans are used. If clinically indicated, a CT scan of the chest or a whole body PET-CT can be done to look for distant metastasis.

Surgical resection, many times with an aggressive approach, is the cornerstone of treatment. For early stage paranasal sinus tumor surgery alone may suffice, and in case there are high risk features like positive margins and others, then adjuvant radiation with or without chemotherapy is to be used. In some patients of even early stages, surgical resection is not possible; in such cases radiation with chemotherapy is a good option.

In patients who are locoregionally advanced, aggressive surgery followed by radiation with chemo are standard. In some cases induction or sequential chemoradiotherapy may be used but the data are not strong in this regard and multidisciplinary discussion should dictate decision making in an individual case.

Paranasal sinuses may give rise to other malignancies as well like adenoid cystic carcinoma, which has an exceptionally high risk of local recurrence. For this reason surgery followed by postoperative radiation therapy is the most rationale treatment. Another not so common type is sinonasal undifferentiated carcinoma, which has a dismal prognosis as local recurrence rates and also those of distant metastasis are very high. Surgery followed by combined chemoradiation offers the best hope for attaining long term response.

Nasal cavity:

Nasal cavity tumors have a varied histology. This chapter will discuss the epithelial malignancies; although lymphoma, melanoma et cetera are commonly found too. The diagnostic workup includes physical examination, endoscopy and imaging studies.

When possible, surgery should be done first and in most of the cases (except T1N0) adjuvant radiation is also to be given. Giving radiation in the preoperative setting should be avoided as it may lead to poor wound healing among other complications.

Nasal cavity is a lymphatic rich area, and patients should receive bilateral elective neck nodal irradiation. Nodes upto and including supraclavicular station should be radiated.

In more advanced cases who are not candidates for upfront surgery, induction chemotherapy can be used to make them resectable. And in cases, final pathology report of whom shows high risk features, radiation therapy should be combined with chemotherapy.

Nasal vestibule:

Now coming to cancers of the nasal vestibule, these are essentially skin cancers. In early stages, surgery and radiation are equally effective and result in high cure rates. In advanced stages, surgery followed by radiation therapy with elective neck irradiation should be done.

CHAPTER 14: HEAD AND NECK CANCERS WITH DISTANT METASTASIS AND RECURRENCE

If head and neck cancers present at early stages, as we have already discussed, the 5-year overall survival and disease free survival figures are high; but even in this subset upto one third or more patients develop recurrence locally or spread distally. And in the case of locally advanced squamous cell carcinoma of the head and neck the aforementioned survival outcomes hover between 30 to 50%; so obviously anywhere between a half to three quarters of the treated patients either don't achieve a complete response, recur or spread to distant sites.

The ultimate prognosis of any such patient is dependent on many factors and the outcome profile can be quite heterogeneous. To make an overly simplistic generalisation, the average overall survival remains dismal, being around 12 months in most instances. On the other hand, some patients present with distant metastatic disease; in these patients the prognosis is dependent upon the sites of metastasis and their numbers. Some of them may fare better than others, thus further adding to the heterogeneity of outcomes. Factors like good performance status, HPV associated cancers and responses to previous or currently ongoing chemotherapy confer good prognosis. Poor performance, prior radiation therapy, age more than 70 years (although the responses are nearly equal in this subset compared to those less than this age, the toxicities are significantly more pronounced) and other coexisting morbid conditions contribute to poor outcomes.

For most patients with distant metastasis and recurrences that are not amenable to local therapies, systemic chemotherapy is the only resort. Just a few years ago, "conventional" cytotoxic chemotherapy used to be the only option. But nowadays immunotherapy has come to the fore and changing paradigms, and so are targeted therapies and small molecule inhibitors.

Patients who have not received systemic chemotherapy previously:

For patients who present with mets or recurrence and have not received chemotherapy previously, cytotoxic chemotherapy is used. Most commonly a combination of two drugs is used, one of which is a platinum compound. Cetuximab can be added to this backbone and results in survival benefit. Another strategy would be to use immunotherapy, but it has not yet been approved in this setting and remains experimental.

When contemplating the first line combination, the historic practice has been to use a platin combined with infusional 5-FU. Around one third of patients are anticipated to show response with this combination but toxicities are many, thus making it a less attractive choice. The next combination is a platin with taxane, the response rates are at least similar to (in many studies better than) the previously mentioned combination with lesser toxicity. Regimens that are commonly used in locally advanced head and neck cancers as induction employ the use of all three of these drugs (cisplatin/carboplatin, 5-FU and paclitaxel/docetaxel); the usage of these drugs in metastatic and recurrent settings does not result in improvement in survival and adds unnecessary toxicity.

EXTREME trial established cetuximab (an EGFR inhibitor) in combination with cisplatin and 5-FU as the most effective regimen that also has a significant survival benefit over cisplatin and 5-FU. There were no significant added toxicities of cetuximab. Another drug belonging to the same category is panitumumab, but it failed to show a benefit in trials done, with only a trend towards increased survival was seen, not reaching statistical significance. Bevacizumab in combination with chemo has been studied and showed improvement in progression free survival, although overall survival improvement didn't reach statistical significance.

In studies published in abstract forms alone, and not yet incorporated in guidelines, immunotherapy has shown promise in patients who have not previously received systemic chemotherapy. Pembrolizumab as a single agent and also in combination with cisplatin and 5-FU showed significant improvements in overall survival compared with cisplatin and 5-FU with or without cetuximab. Further studies are ongoing in this population of systemic therapy naive patients, exploring the role of immunotherapy in the first line.

Patients who have received systemic chemotherapy previously:

Patients, cancers of whom progress after initial systemic chemo given in the curative setting, either as concurrent, induction, sequential or adjuvant; should first be evaluated for the possibility of cure using surgery and/or radiation. If the patient is unfit for undergoing these procedures or the disease is such that it can't be addressed with surgery or radiation then systemic chemo is the only resort. The selection of therapy depends upon patient's performance status, comorbidities and, equally importantly, the response to the initial therapy. If sufficiently enough time has elapsed between the conclusion of initial therapy and recurrence or metastasis (the exact timeline is debated) then the initial chemotherapy regimen may be used again in the hope of attaining the response once again. But if this time has been relatively shorter than another line of therapy is to be used.

In patients who have received platin in the first line and have progressed within a short time, pembrolizumab or nivolumab can be used, alone or in combination with chemotherapy. There is controversy in the usage of immunotherapy is cases with low PD-L1 expression, but even in such cases the toxicities associated with immunotherapy are lesser than conventional cytotoxic chemotherapy. The evidence for supporting the use of pembrolizumab comes from a recently done trial which studied patients who progressed on prior platinum based therapy. These patients were randomized between pembrolizumab as a single agent versus single agent therapy of investigator's choice, including cetuximab, methotrexate or docetaxel. Pembrolizumab was associated with improved survival outcomes and lesser toxicity. Nivolumab also resulted in somewhat similar outcomes.

Many times in practice, due to issue pertinent to reimbursement policies and patient affordability, the use of immunotherapy molecules is not possible. In such cases chemo is to be used. Methotrexate, platins, taxanes, gemcitabine, cetuximab, small molecule tyrosine kinase inhibitors et cetera are options, use of which should fit the clinical situations as a whole; taking into consideration patient's performance status and end organ function. The overall survival on these drugs remains dismal, at around 7-8 months in general.

CHAPTER 15: SECOND PRIMARY MALIGNANCIES

Successful treatment of head and cancer patients is not limited to just the treatment of the primary malignancy (which in itself is no less a feat), but also in surveillance for and treatment of second primary malignancies (SPM). SPM are responsible for the death of up to one third (more in some series) patients of head and neck cancers. The important distinction here is among SPM, recurrences and metastasis. Second primaries may be present at the time of diagnosis of the index cancer, known as synchronous second primaries. This designation of being "synchronous" is valid for second primaries developing within 6 months of the diagnosis of the first head and neck primary. The incidence of SPM is around 2 to 7 percent per year in survivors of head and neck cancers, throughout their lifetime.

The risk factors are continued use of tobacco and

alcohol. Although many SPM develop in people who abstain from these bad habits, it could be attributed to "field cancerization". If radiation therapy was the modality used for a previous head and neck cancer, then its effects on the development are complex. Consensus is that radiation is protective against development of second squamous cell carcinomas, within the field of radiation.

The most frequently used criteria for the diagnosis of SPM were proposed by Warren and Gates, according to these criteria histologic confirmation of malignancy in both the index and secondary tumors must be done, normal mucosa must anatomically separate the two lesions and the possibility of one lesion being a metastatic manifestation of another lesion must be excluded. These criteria seem fine on paper but their practical application is very ambiguous. The distance separating the two lesions is variably described, ranging from 1.5 to 2 cm according to most experts. Also, if a lesion arises at the same site as the index tumor, the time interval that should elapse to call it an SPM versus a recurrence is not agreed upon. Molecular criteria are pursued sometimes but are not validated and confounded by marked tumor heterogeneity.

Most centres use triple (pan) endoscopy for surveillance for SPM. The rationale for this approach is that most of the SPM develop in upper aerodigestive tract which can be picked by panendoscopy. PET-CT scans are being increasingly used but their optimal use and utility is not agreed upon. Once a lesion is found then the aforementioned criteria are applied to establish this new lesion as an SPM.

In general and whenever possible, the treatment of an SPM should follow the internationally accepted guidelines for the site in which it has developed. In other words, an SPM should be treated as any new malignancy affecting that site should be treated, SPM or index. But there are often situations when the treatment plan has to be modified. Like if radiation has already been given to the area from the SPM has now arisen then surgery should be considered first, as reirradiation may not be tolerated well. And if surgery has been done for the index tumor and the SPM has developed in such an area that surgery of it will be excessively morbid then radiation or reirradiation should be opted. The overall prognosis of second primary malignancies is highly heterogeneous and proper guideline driven management increases the chances of attaining long term cure.

CHAPTER 16: SURVIVORSHIP

A cancer survivor is a person who's been diagnosed with cancer. This simple definition highlights the fact that survivorship is a matter of continual appreciation in a person after he's been diagnosed with cancer; it has got nothing to do with the fact whether or not he's been cured of his ailment. But in a more practical way, the discussion of survivorship revolves around those whose disease is in remission, and the general context of discussion are coping with any treatment related side effects, disabilities due to morbid procedures and surveillance for recurrence or second primary.

Surveillance depends on the clinical context and the most rigorous period is the initial two years following treatment and then upto five years. This is an important schedule as almost all recurrences that happen, happen in this period alone, their frequency decreasing with time even in this window.

The optimal schedule of visits in this time frame and beyond is not backed by strong data but the conventional practice and consensus dictates that patients should visit every one to three months for the first year, every two to six months in the second year, every four to eight months during years 3 to 5, and annually beginning five years after the primary treatment.

At each visit detailed history should be taken and a thorough clinical examination is to be performed to discover any new symptom or sign that may point towards a recurrence, second primary or metastasis. In clinical practice often routine imaging studies, like CT scans, are obtained at serial intervals. Not only is this practice not backed by guidelines, it can actually do patients harm; so once the post-treatment scans are normal, routine imaging studies are not to be done, unless there is a clinical suspicion on history or clinical examination. Another very important, vital and potentially harmless part of surveillance is fiberoptic examination. Not only is it informative and safe, it is also relatively easy to perform and cost effective.

Studies have suggested an increased rate of depression and suicide among head and neck cancer survivors. So personal history must be a part of history taking, including details of personal life, major life events, any bad habits and a mental health evaluation; the latter need not be thorough but doing a quick check can sometimes be very fruitful. Patients with history of radiation therapy to the neck should have serum thyroid-stimulating hormone (TSH) levels every 6 to 12 months due to the risk of hypothyroidism. A speech, hearing, and swallowing evaluation and rehabilitation where clinically indicated should be performed.

Head and neck cancer survivors should undergo screening for other cancer, as per the guidelines. Like women should undergo screening for breast cancer, cervix cancer and both sexes for colon cancer and lung cancer et cetera. It is important to mention here that lung cancer shares many etiological agents with head and neck cancer; so many survivors turn out to be screening candidates for lung cancer as well, based on the risk factors established by the lung cancer screening trial.

Maintenance of a healthy lifestyle and avoidance of tobacco and alcohol are inevitable aspects of survivorship. While it goes without saying that smoking is pure evil, but there is some confusion with regard to alcohol usage in head and neck cancer survivors, at least among patients. There are some studies out there, setting limits of "safe" alcohol consumption. These have always been contradictory, but especially in head and neck survivors meta-analysis have clearly shown that consuming even one drink per day leads to an increased risk. So both tobacco **and** alcohol are to be *completely* avoided.

Regular exercise, to the capacity of the individual and being mindful of other comorbidities, is an essential part of survivorship counselling. A Mediterranian diet has proven to be beneficial in many cancer patients and survivors, so it will do no harm to employ this strategy in head and neck cancer survivors as well.

DR. BHRATRI BHUSHAN

Radiation therapy has well known short term and long term effects on oral health, especially dental, mandating evaluation of dental health in survivors. Deterioration of dental and oral health is thought to be secondary to xerostomia, acidification of saliva, demineralization, and defective microvascular circulation. Management includes addressing the problems of xerostomia, mucosal inflammation and dental interventions.

The advent of newer techniques of radiation therapy, namely IMRT has greatly reduced the rates of xerostomia or dry mouth among survivors; but it still remains a major quality of life issue. And in those treated with more conventional methods of radiation delivery, the majority have some degree of xerostomia even years after treatment. It is a cause of continuous distress to the patient and should be addressed promptly.

Complications like osteoradionecrosis, dysphagia, speech difficulty, trismus, lymphedema and neck stiffness are common as well and should be treated by a multidisciplinary team.

Pain can be found in as many as a quarter of the survivors and is a major impediment for a better quality of life. Pain can have multiple pathologies and it depends upon the treatment strategy used as well. Neck surgery can lead to distinct pain "syndromes" like neck and shoulder pain; while radiation can give rise to neuropathic pain patterns.

Medications like gabapentin, carbamazepine, pregabalin, NSAIDs, opioids may have to be used;

HEAD AND NECK CANCER

and so can be cognitive behavioural therapy and advanced pain management services.

A quarter to one half of the survivors may have hearing impairment, due to radiation, cisplatin and their synergistic ototoxicity. Guidelines recommend monitoring for cisplatin induced hearing loss before initiation of treatment (baseline) and before each cycle of treatment and periodically thereafter. Cisplatin induced hearing loss often proves to be permanent, so precautions must be taken and once the hearing loss actually settles later in the course of survivorship then hearing aids should be prescribed.

Peripheral neuropathy is a debilitating complication in long term survivors, as many as three fourth of them face varying degrees of it. Mainly the chemotherapy molecules commonly used are to blame, the effect of cisplatin being cumulative. In patients receiving radiation therapy to the neck, long term autonomic neuropathy is often seen.

Neck muscles and soft tissue get damaged by surgical procedures and radiation therapy also causes fibrosis of these tissues as a stand-alone modality and these effects get accentuated when it's used in combination with surgery. The primary management option once these side effects set in is physiotherapy, although some degree of neck stiffness remain in many survivors.

In a study conducted by Zer et al, there was an increased rate of impaired global neurocognitive functioning among patients who received radiotherapy as part of their definitive treatment planning (38%) at 24 months compared with controls (0%). Further follow-up suggested that head and neck cancer survivors have neurocognitive sequelae up to 2 years after definitive chemoradiotherapy or radiation treatment. Once these cognitive disabilities set in, it's very difficult to overcome them with active interventions. The best cure is prevention, in the form of utilisation of brain sparing techniques like IMRT in every case if feasible.

Studies have reported that patients with head and neck cancer suffer more frequently from mental health conditions and psychological distress than other cancer patients. Diagnosis of SCCHN can subsequently cause patients emotional distress, psychosocial difficulties or psychiatric disorders. Treatment regimens can also impair their physical and psychological well-being, caused by facial disfigurement and physical disability; for example impaired basic functions, such as communication (speaking), breathing, chewing, swallowing, eating (dysphagia) and drinking.

Anxiety and depression can easily develop in these patients as a consequence of the underlying emotional problems the majority of these patients may suffer from. However, despite the fact that these patients may face well-recognized medical, psychological and social challenges, they suffer from both a lack of screening for psychosocial disorders and psychosocial support. Studies report a lack of communication, and information given by oncologists regarding patient emotional and social welfare, and unmet psychosocial needs that can negatively affect many aspects of their care, from compliance to survival.

The lack of support for patients with SCCHN may be responsible for the increased prevalence of depression (22%–57%) and psychological distress compared with patients with other types of cancer. The same is true for the suicide rate (50.5 per 100 000 person years in the United States), which is more than four times the rate of the general population and the overall cancer population.

If the onset of depression is a classic reaction following patient diagnosis with cancer, then patient distress levels would correlate with their understanding of the disease and the realization of how treatment will affect their lives. In fact, studies have reported a correlation between the occurrence (and the level) of anxiety/depression and the level of satisfaction with the information given before treatment. Further studies may identify key areas of improvement, which may be specifically important for patients with SCCHN, such as the provision of information regarding support groups, financial advice, the long-term effects of treatment on the ability to work, physical functioning and quality of life (QoL).

So, patients with head and neck cancers are at a high risk of developing emotional problems at all stages of their disease, and therefore need a support network that closely follows them throughout their journey. Patients do not usually express their emotions spontaneously in front of the oncologist, and there is evidence that patients request less and receive less support from psycho-oncologists. It is imperative that a system is put in place to provide emotional support to SCCHN patients throughout their cancer journey and to encourage them to comply with their ongoing treatment to achieve optimal outcomes. This support could come in the form of one designated health care professional that monitors the patient on an ongoing basis, or as part of an integrated multidisciplinary team management approach. Health care professionals must be aware of this reality and be able to implement psychological interventions during the patient journey. Therefore, for SCCHN patients, the development of psychosocial interventions can be useful in order to improve psychological outcomes and avoid maladaptive coping such as avoiding medical follow-up and continuing their tobacco and alcohol addiction

Second primary malignancy (SPM) represents the leading long-term cause of mortality in patients with head and neck squamous cell carcinoma (HNSCC). Approximately one third of head and neck cancer survivors' deaths are attributable to SPMs, triple the number of deaths that are a result of distant metastases.

SPMs after HNSCC illustrate concepts of field cancerization, in which environmental carcinogens, such as tobacco and alcohol, may induce a field of mucosa afflicted with premalignant disease and may elevate epithelial cancer risk throughout the upper aerodigestive tract. SPMs also provide information regarding common etiologies and epidemiologic trends. The canonical sites of elevated

SPM risk after an index HNSCC are the head and neck, lung, and esophagus (HNLE sites).

As we have already discussed in the section covering surveillance; the detection of second primaries and recurrences are the chief concerns. Adherence to a well formulated follow-up plan is thus imperative for optimal outcomes.

www.ingramcontent.com/pod-product-compliance
Lightning Source LLC
Chambersburg PA
CBHW032025170526
45157CB00002B/860